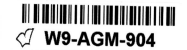
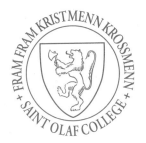

WRONG MEDICINE

DOCTORS,

PATIENTS,

AND FUTILE

TREATMENT **WRONG**

MEDICINE

LAWRENCE J. SCHNEIDERMAN, M.D.
PROFESSOR · DEPARTMENTS OF FAMILY
AND PREVENTIVE MEDICINE AND MEDICINE
· UNIVERSITY OF CALIFORNIA, SAN DIEGO

NANCY S. JECKER, PH.D. ASSOCIATE
PROFESSOR · DEPARTMENT OF MEDICAL
HISTORY AND ETHICS · UNIVERSITY OF
WASHINGTON, SEATTLE

THE JOHNS HOPKINS UNIVERSITY PRESS   BALTIMORE AND LONDON

© 1995 Lawrence J. Schneiderman and Nancy S. Jecker
All rights reserved. Published 1995
Printed in the United States of America on acid-free paper
04 03 02 01 00 99 98 97 96 95   5 4 3 2 1

The Johns Hopkins University Press
2715 North Charles Street
Baltimore, Maryland 21218-4319
The Johns Hopkins Press Ltd., London

ISBN 0-8018-5036-3

Library of Congress Cataloging-in-Publication Data will be found at the
end of this book.
A catalog record for this book is available from the British Library.

Do not try to live forever. You will not succeed.
—George Bernard Shaw, *The Doctor's Dilemma*

CONTENTS

We are fortunate to have had many occasions to present, debate, and shape the ideas expressed in this book. For these invitations, we are grateful to the following persons and institutions:

Thomas Raffin and Ernle Young (Stanford University Medical Center), George P. Baker and Linda and Ezekial Emanuel (Massachusetts General Hospital and the Dana-Farber Cancer Institute), William Donnelly (Edward Hines, Jr., Veterans Affairs Hospital), James Bernat (National Center for Clinical Ethics, Department of Veterans Affairs), Lawrence J. Nelson (Merritt Hospital, Oakland, CA), Sister Sharon Richardt (Daughters of Charity Hospital, Nashville, TN), Angeli O. Oagatep (Kaiser Hospital, Los Angeles, CA), Harold Hassin (Children's Hospital and Health Center, San Diego, CA), Daniel Deykin (Health Services Research and Development Service, Scientific Review and Evaluation Board, Veterans Administration), and Alan Meisel (University of Pittsburgh Medical Center). We also appreciate the invitations from Charles R. Chedister (Riverside Medical Center and Fairview Southdale Hospital, Minneapolis, MN), Sarah Shannon (Seattle Veterans Affairs Medical Center), Richard Winn (Harborview Medical Center, Seattle, WA), Roberta Pagon (Children's Hospital and Medical Center, Seattle, WA), Kaj Johansen (Providence Medical Center, Seattle, WA), Phillip Swanson (University of Washington Medical Center), David Kendall (University of Minnesota, MN), Harris G. Sonnenberg (Unity and Mercy Hospitals, Fridley, MN), Daniel Callahan (The Hastings Center), Alexander Capron (Pacific Center for Health Policy and Ethics, University of Southern California), and James Reitman (Wilford Hall USAF Medical Center). We were also granted forums by Joseph J. Finns (American Geriatrics Society), David A. Bennahum (University of New Mexico School of Medicine), James Walters (Loma Linda University Medical Center), Daniel O. Dugan (El Camino Hospital, Mountain View, CA, and The Park Ridge Center), Nancy N. Dubler (Montefiore Medical Center, New York City), Glen I. Komatsu (Little Company of Mary Hospital, Torrance, CA), Mitsuo Tomita (Kaiser Permanente, San Diego, CA), William Norcross, Marian de

Jesus (The American Academy of Family Physicians), Arthur U. Rivin (Santa Monica Hospital Medical Center), J. Edwin Seegmiller (The Sam and Rose Stein Institute for Research on Aging), Jerry E. Fein (Paradise Valley Hospital, National City, CA), Janet Fleetwood (Medical College of Pennsylvania), Andrew M. Blumenfeld (Kaiser Permanente, Southern California), Steve Daniels (Santa Barbara Cottage Hospital), Kate Christensen (Kaiser Permanente, Northern California), Wayne McCormick (American Association of Home Care Physicians), and Tom Schenkenberg (Department of Veterans Affairs Medical Center, Salt Lake City). The following completes the list of host individuals and institutions: Craig S. Kitchens (University of Florida Medical Center), Stuart Younger (Society for Bioethics Consultation), George Agich and Alain Leplege (First World Congress on Medicine and Philosophy, Paris, France). Also, the Society for Health and Human Values, Indiana University School of Medicine; the Colorado Medical Society; Pacific Physician Services; the American Philosophical Association; the Northwest Network of Ethics Committees; the Eighth National Bioethics Conference, Wahroonga, New South Wales, Australia; the North American Society for Social Philosophy; the American Society of Law and Medicine; and the National Endowment for the Humanities Institute on Medicine and Western Civilization, Columbia University College of Physicians and Surgeons, Center for the Study of Society and Medicine.

We are grateful also to the following for their contributions, ranging from providing stimulating discussions to reviewing chapter drafts: Nancy Dubler, David Burns, Alvin Kalmanson, Don Postema, Haavi Morreim, George Annas, Robert Pearlman, Darryl Amundsen, James Whorton, Edwin Cassem, John Arras, James Walters, James Reitman, Kathy Faber Langendoen, Steve Miles, and Arthur Caplan. We are especially grateful to Albert Jonsen, who from the very beginning helped us explore the ideas presented in this book. Paul Karsten assisted with references.

Finally, we wish to express our boundless gratitude to Sharyn Manning, whose devoted, efficient, skillful organization and attention to detail through the many intricacies of writing this book was indispensable for its completion.

WRONG MEDICINE

CHAPTER 1

ARE DOCTORS

SUPPOSED TO

BE DOING THIS?

Early one January morning in 1983, while driving home from her job in a cheese processing factory, a 25-year-old Missouri woman ran her 1963 Rambler off a country road and landed face down in a ditch. First to arrive on the scene was a state trooper. He examined the young woman and concluded she was dead. Paramedics then arrived—an estimated fifteen minutes after the accident—and immediately set about trying to restore her breathing and heartbeat, which they did after about ten minutes. But the woman never regained consciousness. By then her cerebral cortex, the part of the brain that controls the qualities that made the woman Nancy Cruzan—her thoughts, emotions, behavior, memory, capacity to experience and communicate, in other words, all the activities that make one a unique living person—had been irreversibly destroyed. Only the more primitive part known as the brain stem, which controls heartbeat, respiration, swallowing, and peristalsis, being more impervious to the oxygen deprivation she suffered before cardiopulmonary resuscitation (CPR), only that part of her brain—and those functions—survived. Thereafter, Nancy Cruzan remained unconscious for more than seven years, a condition called permanent vegetative state.[1]

At first, Nancy's family, whose members had become active in a head-injury support group, urged physicians to do everything they could to keep her alive—including surgically implanting a feeding tube into her stomach. But three years later, having witnessed the inevitable grotesque physical changes such patients undergo, including bloating of the face and stiffening contractures of the arms and legs, they asked the doctors to remove the feeding tube so that she could die in peace. Joe Cruzan, a sheet-metal worker, remembered his daughter as a vibrant, independent, cheerful, active woman who loved animals, children, holidays, and the outdoors. "Nancy would not want to live like this," he pleaded, adding that she would be "horrified at her existence now."

But the doctors and the hospital refused to withdraw the feeding tube without a court order, forcing what was from then on the case of *Cruzan v. Director, Missouri Department of Health* to begin its laborious way to the U.S. Supreme Court.[2] The major obstacle to the wishes of the Cruzan family was the Missouri Supreme Court, which declared: "The State's interest is in life; that interest is unqualified."[3] It ordered medical treatment to be continued as long as her body held breath and heartbeat. The court acknowledged that it would have allowed Nancy's tube to be removed if only she had given "clear and convincing" evidence that she would not have wanted to be kept alive in a permanent vegetative state—a contingency beyond the imagination of most people, not to mention a young, vibrant woman in her twenties.

In a highly publicized decision, the U.S. Supreme Court upheld Missouri's right to apply a "clear and convincing" standard for evidence of Nancy Cruzan's wishes. This standard is not defined in any legal textbook or statute; rather, it is "left to the sound discretion of the trial court."[4] But even though the trial court had been persuaded by the parents' testimony that Nancy would have wanted treatment withdrawn, the trial court's decision was overruled by the state supreme court.

After the U.S. Supreme Court's decision, however, a remarkable change occurred in Missouri's view of the matter. Friends of Nancy, whose testimony had never made it to any of the earlier court hearings, reported statements Nancy had made that she would never want to live "like a vegetable" on medical machines. These additional quotations were submitted by the family on remand. Ironically, her friends' testimony appeared to impress the state attorney general more than the statements made by her own parents. But by then, many believe, the state of Missouri, embarrassed by the national outrage at the heartbreaking tragedy, was looking for an excuse to withdraw from the case, which it did in the end, concurring with the trial court that "clear and convincing" evidence had finally been produced and allowing the family's petition to be upheld.

It was not exactly the end, for even after Nancy's feeding tube was removed, carloads of religious zealots descended on the hospital, camped in the parking lots, held prayer vigils, and even tried to force their way in to reattach the tube. But as the Cruzan family said many times, for them Nancy died back in 1983. "The last thing that we could do for her is to set her free,"[5] which they finally accomplished seven years later.

Professor of law George Annas expressed the concerns of many medical ethicists: "The case of Nancy Cruzan provides us with a public warning as to how much control we have already ceded the state over our lives, and how far the state has already gone in redefining the 'life' it seems to 'normalize' and control."[6]

How did medical treatment become such a travesty, such that for the Cruzan family it was not a beneficent healing process but rather an unrelenting scourge? Indeed, Nancy Cruzan's condition, persistent vegetative state, which had not even achieved recognition as a diagnostic entity until 1972, could be regarded as having been caused by medicine itself. Her vegetative state was the consequence of her brain injury, of course, but her *persistent* vegetative state would not have been possible without sustained medical treatment. Today it is estimated that ten thousand to twenty-five thousand such adult patients and four thousand to ten thousand children are being maintained in hospitals and nursing homes around the country.[7] Until the 1970s and '80s these patients rarely were kept alive for long periods of time. What accounts for the difference? It is not that medicine lacked the capabilities—for, ironically, as in the case of Nancy, whose heart, lungs, digestion, and kidneys functioned normally, all it takes is a feeding tube and good old-fashioned nursing care to prevent bedsores and infections.[8] Did financial incentives or fear of litigation suddenly change in the '70s and '80s? Perhaps these are factors—which we will explore in later chapters. But we believe that the principal reason is that maintaining permanently unconscious patients was not considered by society and by physicians to be an appropriate goal of medicine. *Physicians were not supposed to be doing that.*[9]

WHY, THEN, ARE DOCTORS DOING SUCH THINGS?

Hospitals no longer consist of silent wards where patients lie passively waiting to recover from whatever ails them under the watchful eyes of doctors and nurses. Rather, they are bustling, high-technology warrens of specialists. Patients are almost always in motion, aggressively propelled in search of a cure, shunted in and out of elaborately equipped suites providing ultrasound, angiography, fiberoptics, radioactive scanning, computerized axial tomography (CAT) and magnetic resonance imaging (MRI), organ transplants, extracorporeal membrane oxygenation (ECMO), laminar air flow, and the by now old-fashioned intensive care units (ICUs), where patients are connected to ventilators, cardiac pacemakers, and a variety of electronic monitors. The impact of all this technology extends well beyond the innovations themselves; indeed, their most important impact may be on the way doctors think. *Technological imperative* is the term used most often to describe this new way of thinking—if *thinking* is the right word: If a means or instrument or medication exists that can produce an effect, then medicine must use it. In short, the instruments of technology are the focus of attention rather than the patient.

These medical advances, which have brought about incontestable benefits, coincide with the ascending influence of the basic sciences and subspecialties in medical education and practice. Unfortunately, they have caused physicians to fragment their perception of the goals of medicine, leading to an emphasis on the outcomes of discrete parts rather than on the success of the whole.

In contrast, the focus of medical attention throughout the past has always been on the patient. Medical treatments, albeit relatively clumsy, either restored health, or yielded to invalid care, or lost the patient entirely. But the goal of the physician was *at the very least* to restore the patient to some level of conscious awareness and participation in the human community—working, living with loved ones, meeting with friends, watching children and grandchildren play, gossiping, arguing, joking, making love. Today, however, there are so many more intermediary stages between health and death, so many more ways to bring patients from the brink of death back to life, sometimes with only partial recovery of body organs—particularly that most sensitive organ, the brain—that we are now facing ethical problems about the goals of medicine that were unimaginable twenty to thirty years ago. Today patients are being kept alive who cannot experience, much less participate in, the most minimal human activities.

Another new reality about medicine today is that it is no longer a private matter involving only the small circle of patient, family, and physician. Today the circle is more like an arena, and there are many witnesses, participants, even intruders. The Cruzan family, after agonizing discussions in the intimacy of their home, came to the conclusion that medical treatment had failed to bring back their daughter. The goal that they and the doctors had been striving for had not been achieved. They decided therefore to stop medical treatment. But, as it turned out, the decision was not theirs alone to make. Doctors, nurses, hospital administrators, ethicists, lawyers, judges, third-party payers — all demanded a say. The national media picked up the story, and persons whom ethicist Nancy Dubler dubbed "roving strangers,"[10] activists who seek out such cases for the purpose of dramatizing moral or political agendas — these turned the Cruzans' private agonies into a public spectacle.

So, when we question Nancy Cruzan's treatment — Are doctors supposed to be doing these things? — we are actually asking anew the age-old question: What *are* the goals of medicine? Inescapably joined to this question are other questions: Can we as a society agree when treatment fails to achieve the goals of medicine? What are physicians supposed to do and *not* do when treatment fails to achieve the goals of medicine? These are the fundamental questions of medical futility. In answering them we will be examining the doctor-patient relationship as medicine moves into the modern era.

Every day, in our view, the traditions and standards of medicine are being violated by physicians, nurses, and other participants in medical decisions who fail to recognize that the goal of medicine is not and never has been to offer futile treatment. We emphasize that our use of "the goal of medicine" is normative — we believe that often a gap exists between the ends that physicians seek and the ends they *ought* to seek. (Here we invoke the multilayered meaning of the word *ends,* which designates not only goals and purposes but also limits and terminations.)

In short, a desire to restore a vision of medicine's proper ends and reform medical practice is the impetus for this book. Although our central emphasis is to reassert ethical standards for physicians, our arguments have important implications for other health care professionals and other health care fields. And since medicine as a profession is answerable to society, we contend that restoring this vision will require the active involvement of an educated society. Thus, our book is aimed not only at the medical profession and a specialty audience but at the lay public as well.

MEDICAL FUTILITY FROM A HISTORICAL PERSPECTIVE

The view of the goals of medicine and medical futility we present here derives from the long tradition of the profession.[11] Physicians in classical Greece and Rome saw their efforts as assisting nature (*physis*) to restore health. In the treatise titled "The Art," from the Hippocratic corpus, three roles were prescribed for the physician: alleviating suffering in the sick, reducing the violence of their diseases, and refusing to treat those who were "overmastered by their diseases, realizing that in such cases medicine is powerless" (6). Note that the prolongation of life was not considered a goal of medicine.[12]

Long before they made discoveries in the fields of cellular pathology or molecular biology, these scientists of earlier days made careful and remarkably accurate observations of signs and symptoms in their patients to determine the natural course of illness. By empirical experimentation with diet and exercise, herbs and extracts, instruments and splints, they saw themselves as allied with the forces of nature, not with supernatural forces. Indeed, to protect their reputation from accusations of mercenary greed and charlatanism, they forthrightly acknowledged the limits of their skills and duties. "Whenever the illness is too strong for the available remedies," the Hippocratic physician warned, "the physician surely must not even expect that it could be overcome by medicine."[13] The Hippocratic writings further cautioned that a physician should not demand "from an art power over what does not belong to the art, or from nature a power over what does not belong to nature," adding that such ignorance was "allied to madness" (6). Knowing the limits of medicine was regarded as an important measure of a physician's skill in integrating the art of medicine and the power of nature. Thus these early physicians shunned treatments that experience told them were futile and regarded as harmful strenuous efforts to keep an unhealthy patient alive.

Not until many centuries later, in the late Middle Ages, with the rise of Christianity in medieval Europe, did medical practice begin to be dominated largely by religion. During this period, medicine took up "prayer, laying on of hands, exorcisings, use of amulets with sacred engravings, holy oil, relics of the saints and other elements of supernaturalism and superstition."[14] At the same time, the church, which considered abortion, suicide, and euthanasia sins, introduced a new goal in medicine: the prolongation of life.

This new, more expansive view of medicine was reinforced during the scientific revolution of the seventeenth century, when Francis Bacon, for example, defined the goal of science as not merely to "exert a gentle guidance over nature's course" but to "have the power to conquer and subdue her."[15] In other words, scientists began to view science as a power to be exerted *against* nature. Nevertheless, it is important to keep in mind that neither theologians nor scientists, nor for that matter anyone else before the modern era, could ever have imagined life in the many forms in which it comes today, the many states between health and death that are the outcomes of modern medical treatments — for example, Nancy Cruzan's condition, permanent vegetative state.

The classical scholar Darrel Amundsen summarized this evolution and made the following incisive commentary:

> It is well before the advent of modern medicine that physicians were saddled with the expectation that they must do all that they could to cure a patient and they must not desert the patient *in extremis*. Hence, beginning with the late Middle Ages, they were depicted lingering in the background in the death chamber, not able to do anything, but still obligated to be there. The major change since then has been in the increasing capacity of the medical profession to cure disease and prolong life, and the often unrealistic expectations of society that physicians should be able to perform miracles. This has in part resulted from a changed view of nature. Granted, ever since the time of Hippocrates and Plato dispute has intermittently arisen over the question whether the physician works with or against nature in the treatment of illness. Francis Bacon's plea that physicians should seek to prolong life through finding cures for supposedly incurable conditions has blossomed into an attitude that in such a quest it is "man against nature"—the "conquest" of disease involving human ingenuity thwarting nature's purposes.[16]

Later, during the nineteenth century, when medical practice began to profit more conspicuously from the successes of scientific discoveries, not surprisingly it began to pursue more aggressive approaches to treatment. Today we see this combination of religious and scientific impulses survive in casually uttered expressions, such as "life is sacred" and "preserve life at all costs"—high-sounding phrases that have come to dominate medical practice, impelling physicians to pursue even the most futile treatments. But what do we mean by *medical futility?*

DEFINING MEDICAL FUTILITY

We begin our discussion of the ends of medicine by describing, first, what medical futility is not. *Medical futility* does not refer to treatments in a general sense or to patients or to their clinical situations. *Medical futility* refers to a particular treatment applied to a particular patient at a particular time. We also wish to draw attention to the importance of distinguishing among the terms *treatment, therapy,* and *care.* A particular *treatment* (from the root meaning 'to deal with,' literally 'to handle') may be futile, because it fails as *therapy* (from the root 'to heal'). Acts of *care* (from the root meaning 'to feel compassion for') are never futile.

Medicine's goals are clearly to benefit the patient—to restore, to heal ('make whole'). Therefore, they do not include offering treatments that fail to achieve those goals, namely, futile medical treatments. We will devote the remainder of this chapter to presenting and defending a definition of medical futility.

It is important to explain at the outset why a definition of medical futility requires an ethical argument. Unlike definitions of scientific terms, such as *energy* and *mass,* which are part of the discourse of scientists who accept certain scientific theories, the definition of medical futility is not contained in a scientific (or other) theory. Instead, it must rest on a societal consensus that incorporates specific ethical choices—ideas as well as actions. Just as the modern definition of death in terms of "total cessation of brain functioning" reflects society's sense of the meaning of human life, so too whatever definition of medical futility society chooses will reflect its conception of the ethical ends and purposes of medicine.

Some have argued that the whole notion of medical futility is too elusive to define.[17] For example, according to the state of Missouri, Nancy Cruzan's feeding tube was not futile, because it kept her body alive. So we must start out by asking: Is that the goal of medicine — to keep the body, in whatever condition, alive? Is that what we summon up in our mind when we use the word *life* — the irreversibly unconscious body? Don't we rather picture, not a body, but a *person,* someone who is aware of the world around, in touch with it not as a conglomeration of cells and body fluids but as only a specific human being can be — with sensations, thoughts, and emotions? There is no question that the *body* of Nancy Cruzan was not dead. It breathed, pumped blood, digested food, excreted. But was that body the *person,* Nancy Cruzan? Was she in possession of the human capacity to experience her own unique life?

Remarkably, some have tried to reduce the notion of futility to an even more mechanistic and biologically fragmented level. As long as medicine can achieve a physiological effect on any *part* of the body, such as lungs or heart or kidneys, they argue, then treatments such as CPR are not futile.[18] Is this, then, the goal of medicine — to keep an organ system going? Would this satisfy us as a last resort in medical treatment, merely to maintain the flow of air or blood or urine? Most surveys show overwhelmingly that people have other ideas — that past some point in a deteriorating quality of life, well short of merely maintaining organ vitality, they would rather be allowed to die.

Others view futility from the perspective of patient autonomy, arguing that as long as medical treatment can achieve what the patient wants, it is not futile.[19] On first view this would seem a laudable definition of futility. But what if the patient demands surgical removal of unwanted ears, or fingers, or breasts? Or demands that a normal appendix be removed so that he would no longer have to worry that occasional cramps are due to appendicitis? Or demands that doctors carry out cryogenic preservation of her cadaver on the utterly fantastic hope of restoring dead flesh to life? Are there no limits to what medicine owes patients? Clearly there are. Medicine is not a vending machine that dispenses to patients whatever they order regardless of therapeutic efficacy. A physician, for example, is not obligated to provide useless treatment on demand, such as antibiotics for a viral infection or laetrile for cancer. And even if the treatment is *not* useless, physicians are still limited in what they may offer. If a patient's goal is to become a world champion bodybuilder with the aid of steroids, the physician is neither ethically obligated nor legally permitted to comply with the bodybuilder's request. A particularly important limitation, in this era of life as a TV movie of the week, is that the physician does not owe the patient a miracle.

Some bioethicists propose that *futility* refer not just to treatments that cannot benefit patients but also to treatments that provide more harm overall than benefit. The physician–ethicist Howard Brody, for example, argues that anabolic steroids not be provided to the ambitious bodybuilder because, although they may markedly increase physical prowess for a period of ten years, they will in the end lead to deterioration followed by death. By calling such a medicine futile, Brody argues, physicians have a way of keeping intact their professional integrity and the ethical standards of avoiding harm to patients. And so, even if prominent athletic associations declared the use of harmful steroids acceptable by their standards, physicians could refuse such requests on grounds of *their* professional standards.[20]

We have a problem with this definition of futility in that its requirements are too weak; it lets too many treatments qualify as futile. We believe that when the ethical decision amounts to weighing significant *medical* benefits against harms, the responsible adult patient should be allowed to make his or her own decision about treatment. Only when no significant *medical* benefit can come from using a particular intervention does it become the physician's responsibility to inform the patient that the treatment will not be offered.

In our view, the anabolic steroid is futile not because it harms patients down the road but because it does not provide any medical benefits to patients in the first place. After all, enhancing athletic prowess is not a medical goal; rather, medicine is concerned with restoring health and healing the patient. Giving an athlete large doses of steroids certainly does not make a sick person well, nor does it rehabilitate a handicapped person to a level of ordinary functioning. There was a notorious time in recent history when Nazi doctors aspired to make a super-race by selectively breeding those they thought possessed superior qualities and exterminating those they thought lacked such qualities. But this goal, which violates the fundamental duty of beneficence to every patient, never has been part of the historical tradition of ethical medicine. Nor does the ethical practice of medicine embrace such a goal today.[21]

It should be clear, then, that the above definitions of the goals of medicine and medical futility are unsatisfactory. The challenge we face is to provide a useful and persuasive alternative definition that not only serves at the patient's bedside but also is acceptable to society at large. For without the informed agreement by an educated and active public, current medical practices will continue unabated, with all the irrationalities and painful and costly habits unchanged.

By proposing a definition of medical futility, rather than simply a description or example of futility, we hope to provide the necessary and sufficient conditions for a medical intervention falling under the term. At present, the everyday understanding of futility in the medical setting is often vague, and determining futility is often problematic. By saying that the present usage of *futility* is vague, we mean that many people who use this term do not fully understand its meaning; at present, the term lacks a clear meaning. Yet a vague term can become clearer when it is more fully specified. For example, *obscenity* is sometimes a vague term. Its meaning becomes clearer, however, when the Supreme Court decides that certain record albums contain obscene lyrics, thus providing substantive information about the meaning of the term. This is analogous to how we intend to provide a definition of futility. However, unlike the legal definition of obscenity, the definition of futility we propose must ultimately be accepted and validated by health professionals and the public at large.

We will start therefore with a preliminary general definition of medical futility. *Medical futility means any effort to provide a benefit to a patient that is highly likely to fail and whose rare exceptions cannot be systematically produced.* Note first that this definition has a quantitative component ("highly likely to fail") and a qualitative component ("benefit to the patient"). Note also that the focus of the effort is the patient (derived from the Latin word for 'to suffer'), not some organ or physiological function or body substance. Nor is the patient merely any person who has some capricious desire, but a specific kind of person, one who is in particular need of the medical skills and judgment of a physician to alleviate or prevent suffering. Note also that what is provided is a benefit, not an effect. There is an important difference. Medicine is capable of an enormous range of effects that once were unimaginable—adding and subtracting body chemicals, increasing and reducing circulating blood cells, destroying cancer cells, restoring heartbeat, replacing kidney function, killing bacteria, subduing viruses and fungi, to name a few. But these effects are of no benefit to the patient unless the patient is capable of appreciating them. The sad fact is that medical treatments could have produced a multitude of effects on the unconscious Nancy Cruzan, but she was incapable of appreciating any of them. Thus, in our view, all the treatments aimed at Nancy Cruzan, because they provided no benefit, were futile, and health professionals had no business attempting them.

In reviewing the Cruzan case, it is important that we make clear the reasons underlying our judgment that it is futile to provide life-sustaining treatment to Nancy Cruzan. All patients with complete and permanent loss of consciousness, such as permanent vegetative state, lack a necessary feature of being a person. For, regardless of widely different conceptions of personhood, almost everyone agrees that personhood requires consciousness and self-awareness. If permanently unconscious patients are not persons, it follows that health professionals have no business attempting treatments to keep them alive; for the subject of medical treatment is not the biological body but the suffering patient. Although ethical considerations, such as respect for the patient's dignity and compassion for the family, may lead doctors to provide other forms of treatment, such as anticonvulsants or hygienic care, they are under no duty to offer life-sustaining treatments. Indeed, in subsequent chapters of this book we will make the case that physicians not only are not obligated to offer futile treatments, they *should* not offer futile treatments.

Now it might mistakenly be argued that the mere fact that a permanently unconscious individual is a living member of our species suffices to show that that individual is a "person" and therefore is an appropriate subject of medicine. However, it is important to distinguish carefully between "person," which carries moral connotations, and "human being," which is used in its descriptive biological sense. As philosophers use the term, *person* refers to a being, potentially of any species, who possesses the qualities that are necessary and sufficient for possessing fundamental moral rights, including a right to life. Hence, if permanently unconscious patients are not persons, then by definition they lack a right to life, and are not owed the medical means necessary to stay alive. Once again we point out that neither late medieval theologians nor seventeenth-century scientists who advocated life-prolongation were familiar with living human beings who were not also conscious (even if severely impaired) persons. Nor were they likely to have imagined the notion of "life" that can be preserved in such a discordant state by present-day technology.

It is worth noting that some who agree that human beings in a permanent vegetative state lack the moral qualities necessary to qualify as moral persons, with a right to life, will argue that all forms of human life (both personal and nonpersonal) possess intrinsic value. For them, even nonpersonal forms of human life possess special value (or, in religious terms, "sanctity" or "sacredness"), and therefore there is some merit to preserving them.

We sympathize with the humane impulse behind this argument, but respond that even if one thought that human life in any form was intrinsically valuable, it hardly follows that it is *medicine*'s job to attempt to preserve all forms of human life. Medicine's focus has never been (and should never become) the biological organism as such, but is the suffering *person* (i.e., patient). Thus, even though physicians may have a responsibility to treat human life—from the earliest stages of conception to brain death—with dignity and respect, only persons are proper subjects of life-sustaining medical treatment. To draw an analogy, nearly everyone agrees that a brain-dead individual is a past person, and as such the physical remains should be treated with respect; however, a brain-dead individual is no longer seen as a *patient* or an appropriate subject of life-sustaining *medical* treatment. In other words, even though a brain-dead individual continues to be a living human organism, it is not a living human person. This marks a crucial turning point in how medicine views it. Once a patient meets the criteria for brain death, medical apparatus, such as respirators and artificial fluid and hydration, are withdrawn. Likewise, we are arguing that an individual in a permanent vegetative state is a past person, whose biological remains should be treated with dignity and respect. However, it should not be medicine's task to use the means at its disposal to keep the physiological processes of such an individual running.

FURTHER DEFINING MEDICAL FUTILITY: ITS QUANTITATIVE ASPECT

One thing every medical student learns is "never say never." This is the problem of uncertainty in medicine. Quantitative probabilities can never be precisely determined. Clinical circumstances are so complex that one can never be absolutely certain of the outcome. Indeed, philosophers since David Hume have pointed out that the very notion of causality is suspect. As Hume noted, we never directly observe the "causal glue" that connects two events. Instead, "the mind goes beyond what is immediately present to the senses" to infer a causal relationship.[22] The contemporary philosopher Karl Popper emphasizes that science can never produce knowledge that is certain. Even after we fail a million times to resuscitate a cadaver—drawing the not unreasonable conclusion that the dead cannot be revived—how do we know the next effort will not result in success? It would take only one success to falsify the conclusion drawn from all the previous experiences.[23] In medicine, for example, we have no way of knowing with certainty that a treatment causes an effect to occur in the body. We observe only that on numerous occasions the application of this kind of treatment precedes bodily changes. We *infer,* on the basis of probability, that the treatment is the responsible (causal) agent. It is important to make this point clear: Medical practice almost never achieves certainty; rather, it depends on empirical clinical experience. Physicians prescribe specific drugs and dosages because such treatments have been observed to achieve beneficial effects (over unwanted side-effects) sufficiently often in the past that they feel confident these practices will work in the future. But each patient represents a new challenge—will the particular drug and dosage work on this particular patient in this particular circumstance? Uncertainty lurks in the shadow of every medical decision.

Today, as more and more therapeutic options have become available, this struggle with uncertainty has led to a paradox, a kind of paralysis of action. If the physician can never be absolutely certain, then isn't the physician obligated to do anything and everything that might conceivably work? This paralysis of action expresses itself in a relentless momentum. Once high-technology machines are started—which might conceivably work—they are almost impossible to stop. But the world is full of tales of miraculous events, up to and including the raising of the dead. Physicians have never been obligated—or even expected—to reproduce all the miracles of mythology. That is what we mean by "rare exceptions [that] cannot be systematically produced." At most, physicians can do their best to "assist nature" in the real world. To overcome this paralysis of action in the face of uncertainty, we pose the following common-sense question: *Since we can never say never, can we agree that if a treatment has not worked in the last 100 cases, it would be "reasonable" to conclude that it is futile?* We propose this then as our specific and practical definition of the quantitative aspect of medical futility.

Although we have presented a specific proposal, we recognize that people may disagree about exactly where the threshold for futility should lie. For example, some may think that waiting for 100 failures before acknowledging a treatment's futility sets the threshold too low. However, the important consideration is that all would probably agree with our more general claim that *at some point* the likelihood of medical success is so poor that attempting to achieve it is futile.

But what about those who do not agree, who refuse to accept any notion of futility? For example, what about the person who argues: If I'm willing to pay for it, why can't I have life support for my child's permanent vegetative state as long as I want? Or what if a religious group expresses the belief, based on a biblical precedent, that resurrection is possible and demands that the dead bodies of its adherents be preserved with mechanical ventilation, cardiac stimulation, and intravenous fluids?

In response, we would first point out that physicians' professional responsibilities prohibit them from providing a treatment solely because someone is willing to pay for it. As we will emphasize often in this book, the goals and limits of medicine are not determined merely by money. Medicine, as a profession, is distinguished by the goal of healing patients. If it were to be practiced solely to satisfy the whims of those who would pay, the ethics of medicine would become indistinguishable from those of the "oldest profession." Therefore, any proposal to permit medical consumers to obtain different levels of treatment above a "decent minimum" depending on their willingness to pay still must remain within the limits of the appropriate goals of the health care profession: medically beneficial care. And just as no health-care plan allows physicians to provide steroids to athletes willing to pay for the drugs, no plan should authorize physicians to provide futile treatments to those patients willing to pay higher premiums.

As for the second objection to futility based on religious beliefs, we will deal with this subject at greater length in Chapter 7. Here we will briefly note, however, that in our pluralistic society, religions with specific beliefs that impinge on medical practice are not free to impose those beliefs on others, although they are free to form their own medical provider systems that provide and pay for such practices.

Interestingly, a consensus already seems to be forming in the medical community about the application of our quantitative notion of futility. In the past few years, studies have begun to appear evaluating CPR in a variety of patients, ranging from very low-birth-weight babies to elderly patients to patients with metastatic cancer to patients rushed to the emergency department after experiencing irreversible cardiac arrest outside the hospital. Independently, the research physicians at different medical centers came to the same conclusion: Even though CPR occasionally produced a few hours or even a few days more of life in the hospital, the procedure was futile, since it failed to result in hospital discharge in more than about 1 in 100 of these patients.[24] Thus, neither the probability nor the quality of the outcome was regarded as fulfilling the goals of medicine.

FURTHER DEFINING MEDICAL FUTILITY: ITS QUALITATIVE ASPECT

In *The Republic,* Plato wrote: "For those whose lives were always in a state of inner sickness Asclepius [a mythical demigod-physician] did not attempt to prescribe a regimen . . . to make their life a prolonged misery." And "a life of preoccupation with illness and neglect of work isn't worth living."[25]

Unfortunately, as our technological skills have become more powerful and the technological imperative more compelling, "prolonged misery" has afflicted many of those who fall by the wayside while hoped-for miracles are being pursued. The misery, however, and the costs and suffering involve not only the treatment failures. What about those for whom treatment is considered a success? In the past, a successful treatment was not so dubious or problematic. Inevitably, the patient appreciated it as a benefit. Can we say that of Nancy Cruzan, as she lay in her unconscious state, with her cerebral cortical tissue atrophied and replaced by fluid? Nancy experienced nothing — certainly no benefit from her survival. Nor would she ever. Thus, we must consider a qualitative aspect to medical treatment. In other words, we must distinguish between an *effect* and a *benefit*.

As we have already said, we believe that treatment of a patient such as Nancy Cruzan in permanent vegetative state is by definition futile because she is incapable of experiencing, much less appreciating, anything that is being done to her. We would argue also that the goal of medicine is not to keep people alive in the intensive-care unit (ICU), where they are *preoccupied* (to use Plato's word) with treatment and can do nothing else with their life. Such patients are there because they require constant and close attention as well as immediate access to physicians, nurses, and technicians who can diagnose and treat medical crises. They cling to life by machines designed to blow oxygen into their lungs, machines designed to monitor body fluid balance and blood chemicals, and still other machines designed to sound shrill warnings while initiating and controlling heartbeat and responding to shock. When they were developed in the 1960s, ICUs were intended to be only temporary havens for desperately ill patients who would be expected either to die or to recover. But today, ICUs have become a kind of purgatory for many patients who remain for months and months on the brink of death before succumbing to their illness. Such patients totally depend on intensive medical care for survival — in the ICU. Is this a goal of medicine, to sustain life in the ICU? We believe not.

Thus, our specific and practical definition of the qualitative aspect of medical futility: *If a patient lacks the capacity to appreciate the benefit of a treatment, or if the treatment fails to release a patient from total dependence on intensive medical care, that treatment should be regarded as futile.*

Again, not everyone may agree with the threshold we have

chosen for qualitative futility. For instance, some may urge that a life-saving treatment be regarded as futile if the patient will not survive to hospital discharge. Others may accept our more conservative view that life-saving measures on behalf of a patient who is confined to a hospital bed are not necessarily futile. Despite these specific disagreements, we believe that everyone can agree with our more general idea that *at some point* the quality of medical outcome may become so poor that it is futile.

Admittedly, our own position is conservative, for, as we have already noted, a medical consensus seems to be forming that if a treatment doesn't lead to discharge from the hospital, it should be regarded as futile. In any case, it appears that physicians are beginning to reevaluate not only their duties and obligations but also their limits. This is an important first step. But ultimately, society at large will have to express agreement clearly: The ends of medicine lie not with mere biological survival nor with the patient imprisoned within machines and tubes. At the very least, the ends of medicine require providing the patient with the capacity to participate in the human community. And though this level of participation can be minimal, common sense would dictate that it does not refer to insensate bodies or patients irrevocably immersed in a hospital's life-support machinery. We strongly advocate patient autonomy and the right to make medical treatment decisions over a wide qualitative range—and there are many noteworthy examples of people who have achieved remarkable satisfaction despite severe physical or mental handicaps—but we draw a line between patients' rights to choose their own quality of health and life and the medical profession's obligations to achieve those ends. Limits should be clearly stated: Patients can demand of medicine help in maintaining any quality of life they like so long as that life is not irreversibly unconscious or confined to the ICU—for these are beyond the goals of medicine. On the other hand, we wish to emphasize a point we have already made: A particular *treatment* may be futile, but *care* is never futile; nor is a *patient* ever futile. The second, qualitative dimension of futility provides a sufficient condition for a treatment counting as futile. In other words, if an intervention meets this criterion, that is all that is needed to show that it is futile.

Taken together, the quantitative and qualitative standards we

CHAPTER 2

T IS HARD

Y NO

Our medical ethics consultations take many forms. They range from nocturnal phone calls from resident physicians worried about the legal risk of accepting a patient's request not attempt resuscitation (DNAR) order, to bedside discussions ntensive care unit (ICU) with distraught or resigned patients, ed and lengthy conferences involving every combination of families, doctors of varying specialties, nurses, psycholo- cial workers, lawyers and hospital administrators. Inevitably, emotions become interwoven with philosophical reflections, s in the human repertoire that moral philosophers have tra- ly tried to keep apart. By the time we are called to assist in al decision, there is rarely an obvious "right" answer. The sit- s beyond a simple fix. Instead, the ethics consultant, together e health care team, faces options that are charged with irra- opes at best, intolerable outcomes at worst. And yet so often, ime we are called, decisions have already been made to press certain treatments, despite a general acknowledgment that er choice would have been an entirely different approach. es this happen? Why is it so hard to say no to treatments that rly providing no benefit and are only prolonging suffering? cia M. was a 14-year-old girl with leukemia. Her disease had l several times over the past few years despite chemotherapy. ough Alicia was legally a minor, the medical team was im- that she had a full understanding of her illness and treat- As her condition took a decisive turn for the worse, she be- express a preference for narcotics and other measures that maximize comfort as opposed to chemotherapy, antibiotics nsfusions, treatments aimed at prolonging her life. But her , avid bodybuilders and physical fitness buffs, kept urging to give up. They persuaded her and the medical team to at- bone marrow transplantation despite the low odds of suc- his treatment required ablating her immune system first with dy irradiation and chemotherapy. Her postoperative period

propose for medical futility provide the necessary and sufficient condition for medical futility. Each criterion is sufficient by itself to confer medical futility, yet meeting one or the other of these criteria is necessary.

In Chapter 4 we stress the importance of continuing to offer comfort care to the patient and emotional support to the family after futile interventions are stopped. In Chapter 5 we distinguish between withholding treatments on the basis of futility and withholding treatments on the basis of rationing. The medical profession does not owe every treatment imaginable; but until society establishes a policy of rationing that applies just limits to medical treatments, the medical profession owes to every patient, in whatever condition, a choice of any treatment that can provide medical benefits.

Ironically, there is an unexpectedly positive consequence to forcing physicians and patients to acknowledge medical futility. Instead of continuing the useless repetition of unsuccessful treatments, physicians will be spurred to search for more beneficial treatments. An honest acknowledgment of futility, in our opinion, will make medical progress and discovery more likely rather than less likely.

THE MYTHICAL POWER OF FUTILE TREATMENT

Until now we have refrained from the obvious, that is, stating the dictionary meaning of futility. In the *Oxford English Dictionary* the word is defined as "leaky, vain, failing of the desired end through intrinsic defect." The word derives from the ancient *futtilis,* a pot, wide at the top and narrow at the bottom, that was used in religious ceremonies on behalf of Ceres, the goddess of fertility, and Vesta, the hearth goddess. Because of its narrow base, the *futtilis* tipped over whenever it was filled. Although the *futtilis* was useless for everyday tasks, as a religious vessel it played a powerful role in mythic drama. The philosopher Don Postema asks, "Can a medical treatment similarly be useless from one point of view, but have mythic significance from another perspective? What cultural meanings do futile therapies carry?"[26]

Postema goes on to point out that Sisyphus has always been seen as a symbol of futility, being condemned to Hades to eternally roll a rock up a hill, only to see it roll down again. "However," Postema adds, "Albert Camus in the 'Myth of Sisyphus' takes the character and life of Sisyphus as an emblem for the modern age, a hero in an absurd world. Sisyphus is a tragic figure because he is conscious of his task; he knows that what he is doing is futile, yet he persists in its performance."[27]

Postema thus reminds us of the importance of symbols. We must ask, does the pursuit of futile treatment serve some need of patients for heroic action? Does it provide some deeply felt cravings in an antiheroic age? Does it offer a magical alternative to the mundane world of cause and effect? One of the realities of contemporary society is that medicine has for the most part replaced religion as a source of spiritual meaning and consolation and miraculous expectation. Many treatments, such as CPR, have become rituals in the mind of the public, conveying religious and mythical power. Is it in answer to these deep spiritual needs that patients and families sometimes demand futile treatments? Are these life-saving treatments misguidedly taken as measures of caring and compassion? Images of abandonment are frequently heard and words such as *starvation* and *neglect* used to describe dying patients who are not connected to intravenous lines or gastrostomy tubes or ventilators or assailed with CPR. Sadly, however, futile interventions are not good ways to promote caring and compassion. Often they are obstructive and harmful. All too often, they make a mockery of caring by substituting invasive procedures for human communication and touch, only adding to patient discomfort in the terminal stages of disease.

In pursuing our concept of futility throughout this book, we hope we have not lost sight of the spiritual needs of a modern society that for the most part has lost faith in religion. Good physicians often call upon priests, ministers, rabbis, and other spiritual leaders for help in caring for their patients. But the reverse also has occurred, particularly in the last few decades when patients and families have come to look for miracles from medicine and science rather than from religious sources. In the past when people sought a miracle, they went to church and prayed to God. Now they go to the hospital and demand it of the doctor.

Medicine has not been an unwilling collaborator in this deception, taking advantage of the public's infatuation with "miraculous breakthroughs," "miracle drugs," and other hyperbolic claims. It was

inevitable that medicine would be held to acc uncommon for members of the clergy and ju support highly emotional (and often well-p patients and families for outcomes that are b medical practice, not to mention science. H ethicist Albert R. Jonsen reminds us:

> The public and physicians alike are affected b ing and life sustaining technologies. But the tive when they reach beyond the reality. Th does have real but limited efficacy. Refusal to ture of medicine's efficacy is to honor the sy ity. It deceives patients and the public rather enhancing their autonomy. Far from depriv the appropriate invocation of futility reveal persons have when they seek help from mo

It is this distortion of the goals of medicine t Nancy Cruzan.

As David Rothman, a professor of soci argues, the most important issues today ha budget or with concern for the common wi tion of futility, a desire to prevent pain, and evitable."[29]

In the next chapter we will explore wl the inevitable and say no to futile treatment the approach we will take throughout the k ing opposing perspectives, we clearly inten own. Like law professor Ronald Dworkin, v *Dominion,* addresses abortion and euthanas for pursuing an extended argument rather hands a bland on-the-one-hand-on-the-o we hope that the reader will find "an exar genre: an argumentative essay that engag begins with, and remains disciplined by, a political importance."[30]

for
in
to
pat
gis
inte
acti
diti
a m
uati
witl
tion
by t
on
the
Why
are

relap
Even
press
ment
gan
woul
and t
paren
her n
temp
cess.
total

was punctuated by several near-fatal episodes of shock and sepsis. Finally, she developed large areas of open, painful and easily contaminated skin wounds and required a ventilator to assist her breathing.

Prodded by the nurses, the doctors finally agreed among themselves that continuing ventilator treatment in these circumstances was futile and that Alicia had no realistic chance of overcoming her present condition. All they were doing was prolonging her suffering. After consulting with one of us to gain reassurance about ethics and the law, the physician in charge of Alicia's care presented the facts to the family. He strongly urged that Alicia be kept comfortable with sedation and narcotics and be allowed to die without any further efforts at resuscitation or life-prolongation. The parents resisted at first, then agreed. But as they sat by their sleeping daughter's bedside and watched her breathing become weaker and more irregular, they abruptly changed their minds and demanded that vigorous measures be reinstituted to treat her faltering heart and blood pressure and assist her breathing and combat infection. So fiercely did the parents express themselves that the doctors relented and resumed aggressive measures at life-prolongation, placing Alicia back on the ventilator and starting IV medications to stimulate her heart, raise her blood pressure, and combat infection. But these measures served only to keep her alive and miserable three more days. For months afterwards, in the dining room, in the nursing stations and corridors, in fact almost everywhere doctors and nurses gathered, the young girl was the subject of anguished discussions. Why had they let that happen? Why had it been so hard to refuse the demands of Alicia's parents for treatments all the health providers had come to agree were futile?

In this chapter we will briefly present some of the reasons we have encountered in our clinical ethics work. In later chapters we will discuss them in more detail. Some of the factors are inextricably linked to the human psyche; some reflect our contemporary medical culture and the training of physicians and nurses; others arise out of "real world" legal and political considerations.

Human beings resist death. This fact is so self-evident that we consider it unnatural—pathological—when a person seeks to die. A physician, confronted by a patient expressing suicidal thoughts, would most likely make a diagnosis of severe depression, seek to assess the immediate risk, and either attempt treatment or call upon a psychiatrist to manage the patient. Physicians are even granted legal authority in most states to take control of patients who are judged to be suffering from a mental illness and likely to harm themselves, and hospitalize them against their will. This is evidence that society assumes that normal, healthy people would resist death and only deranged people would not. Indeed, preferring death over life is seen not only as irrational but as sinful by many segments of society. Yet a patient might *wish* to live, but not in an intolerable state. Thus, one reason why it is so hard to say no to futile treatment, is that since society's life-protecting propensities are so strong, its first impulse—and the impulse of medical providers—is to keep life going at all costs. In the case of Alicia's parents, this attitude contained an even more powerful component. They took pride in challenging their bodies, and experienced pleasure and enhancement of their self-image when they could triumph over pain and physical limits. For them, life seemed to possess even greater value when it was death-defying. Although this heroic view of life is in many ways admirable, it became a terrible curse when projected onto another human being, their daughter, whose illness and suffering had led her to a different view of life.

Human beings have difficulty accepting their humanity. Philosopher Martha Nussbaum suggests that the difficulty we have in accepting the limits of our mortality is that such acceptance *requires* a kind of heroism. In her rich and perceptive essay, "Transcending Humanity," she draws attention to the moment in the wanderings of the mythological Odysseus when he rejects Calypso's offer to settle down. She had tempted him with immortality and ageless love. Odysseus acknowledges that his wife, Penelope, is far beneath the beautiful goddess in form and stature: "She is mortal," he admits, "you are immortal and unaging."[1] Yet, even so, the long-suffering sailor opts to continue his voyage, thus choosing "not only risk and difficulty, but the certainty of death; and not only death, but the virtual certainty that he will at some time lose what he most deeply loves, or else will cause, by his own death, great grief to her. . . . He is choosing the whole human package: mortal life, dangerous voyage, imperfect mortal aging woman. He is choosing, quite simply, what is his: his own history" (366).

Referring to the ancient Greek concept of hubris, Nussbaum goes on to say,

> There is a kind of striving that is appropriate to a human life; and there is a kind of striving that consists in trying to depart from that life to another life. This is what *hubris* is — the failure to comprehend what sort of life one has actually got, the failure to live within its limits (which are also possibilities), the failure, being mortal, to think mortal thoughts. Correctly understood, the injunction to avoid hubris is not a penance or denial — it is an instruction as to where the valuable things *for us* are to be found. (381)

In medicine, hubris tempts patients and physicians to strive to exceed medicine's limits and ask for everything, even the impossible. Yet when a humanly meaningful life is no longer possible, the better course is to follow Odysseus's model: to choose our own history with humility and dignity.

Physicians have difficulty accepting the limits of their power. Physicians, too, suffer from a corresponding hubris. As the ethicist Daniel Callahan observes, the modern era of medicine has transformed death from a biological or natural evil to a moral evil and medical failure, as though an amendment had been added to the physician's Hippocratic Oath: "If we do not use our newly available technologies to save lives, we can be held accountable for the loss of those lives."[2] This transformation in our attitudes toward death occurs from the very beginning by medical education and the socialization of medical students, then is reinforced every day by medical practice, which takes credit for both saving and failing to save life. Rather than regarding death as our common and inevitable fate, or locating our own mortality within nature's cycle of birth and death, medicine has come to view death as its enemy to conquer. Rather than admitting the possibility that certain states of existence are worse than death, medicine tends to imagine that death always represents the worst kind of "evil empire."

These assumptions must be examined anew in order to make room for the idea of medical futility and a more realistic appraisal of medicine's limits. Medicine's basic commitment is not to life in any

form, but to the patient, the "suffering person." Therefore, a patient's
death is not necessarily a failure to achieve medicine's goals. Indeed,
a "good" death, as viewed by the physician-ethicist Howard Brody,
should be "hailed as a medical success story." Brody reminds his colleagues that "all our patients eventually die, and it is wrongheaded to
see death itself as a sign of medical failure. Rather, we should acknowledge failure when the ravages of disease or ill-constructed
medical interventions produce a 'bad' death."[3]

The physicians treating Alicia's leukemia had at their command
a vast array of treatment possibilities, including powerful (and toxic)
chemicals that destroyed her leukemia cells (along with many other
kinds of cells), and antibiotics to attack viruses, bacteria, and fungi.
They even had a capability that a few decades ago was no more than
a scientific hope based on promising experiments in mice—a technology that made it possible to replace the very marrow in her bones.
Because of the seemingly limitless powers at their disposal, Alicia's
physicians probably grew accustomed to the idea that they always
had something more they could offer. Rather than encouraging humility, which the moral philosopher Karen Lebacqz calls "a sense of
one's limits . . . one of the goods internal to the practice of health
care,"[4] their technological skills, instruments, and medicines may
well have lured the physicians into a delusion of omnipotence. This
sense of power resembles that of a ganglord carrying a concealed
gun. Admitting the limits of their power leads them to feel not
merely diminished, but devoid of their very identity. The hardest
thing for the ganglord would be to go out in the streets without his
weapon. The hardest thing for some physicians is to face the family
of a dying patient without some new technological offering, in
short, to be honest. The kindest approach would be to acknowledge
that there is nothing more to do to save their loved one's life and add,
"Now we will do everything to help her to live out her last days and
die with as much comfort and dignity as possible." Sadly, it is much
easier for many physicians simply to attempt a new futile treatment,
making a show of intense commitment to the patient as a way of convincing observers that they are using their powers to the fullest.

Not surprisingly, it was the nurses, rather than the physicians,
who were the first to show genuine understanding of Alicia's condition. By her bed constantly and perceiving that her drawn-out exis-

tence would be wracked with pain and suffering, the nurses realized that continuing to apply life-saving interventions would be a cruel and uncaring response. Perhaps they saw that the respirator's primary goal had become one of comforting the family and the physicians, not the patient.

We would argue further that forcing Alicia to be entirely preoccupied with receiving medical treatment, so that she could not even communicate meaningfully with family and friends, condemned her to live her last weeks of life banished from the human circle of family and community. In the past such a banished existence was imposed as punishment for capital crimes and considered worse than death. Perhaps Alicia's nurses recognized better than her physicians that a life apart from the web of relationships and projects that fasten a person to the human social world was in its own way a state worse than death. Such a state of banishment, whether it consists of unremitting pain and suffering or perpetual unconsciousness, cannot be regarded as a beneficent goal of medicine.[5]

Everyone has struggled so hard, we can't give up now. Sarah J. was a 7-month old girl with congenitally abnormal lungs who received a lung transplant at one of the country's leading medical centers. For months following the surgery, Sarah never left the hospital as the doctors struggled to keep the child alive, despite increasing evidence that the congenital condition affecting her lungs involved other organ systems as well. Soon it became apparent that the child was doomed to die, but because the physicians had worked so hard, and the child (and the child's parents) had suffered so much, no one had the heart to call it quits. Only when a military reassignment forced the parents to move and transfer the child to a different hospital were they put in the hands of new physicians who felt no such emotional burden. To these physicians the futility of continuing with various life-preserving interventions was clearly apparent. A conference was arranged with the family, physicians, nurses and an ethics consultant. Painful facts were laid out and discussed frankly and sympathetically. Confronted with this fresh approach, the parents reevaluated their feelings and soon agreed to let their daughter die without any further suffering.

This problem with the intense and sometimes rocky course of

organ transplantation is not uncommon. Post-transplant care involves the most sophisticated weapons in the technological arsenal, and can be an emotional roller coaster, with miraculous survival waiting at one end and death buried within tubes and machinery in an isolated, laminar flow room at the other. Physicians, patients and their families become locked in a mutual dependency, relentlessly pursuing more and more desperate and futile measures to keep the patient alive—including even repeated efforts at transplantation—because of the momentum that developed. Yet the facts are harsh. If a first heart or liver or lung transplant fails, a second effort in the wake of the failure has a much poorer chance of success.[6] Others waiting desperately for their first chance at such organs would almost certainly do better. But when asked about the apparent irrationality of performing repeat organ transplant operations despite the sharply reduced odds of success, surgeons will almost always point out how emotionally difficult it is to "abandon" a patient once the process has begun. "Everyone struggled so hard, we just couldn't give up."

Why is everyone miraculously rescued but me? In an eloquent passage from her novel *Death Comes for the Archbishop,* Willa Cather described the "solemn social importance" of death in an earlier era:

> In those days, even in European countries, death had a solemn social importance. It was not regarded as a moment when certain bodily organs ceased to function, but as a dramatic climax, a moment when the soul made its entrance into the next world, passing in full consciousness through a lowly door to an unimaginable scene. Among the watchers there was always the hope that the dying man might reveal something of what he alone could see; that his countenance, if not his lips, would speak, and on his features would fall some light or shadow from beyond. The "Last Words" of great men, Napoleon, Lord Byron, were still printed in gift-books, and the dying murmurs of every common man and woman were listened for and treasured by their neighbours and kinsfolk. These sayings, no matter how unimportant, were given oracular significance and pondered by those who must one day go the same road.[7]

Today, patients who learn they have an incurable illness are more likely to feel only isolation and betrayal. All around them, it seems, another lucky soul is displayed on the evening news, having been rescued from the brink of death by miraculous drugs, virtuoso operations, and the latest scientific discoveries. Small wonder that many of those who expect no such triumphant outcomes feel ignored and cast aside amidst the celebrations of modern medicine. To die is perceived not as something inevitable, a moment to be treasured, but as an avoidable mishap — if only the person had the strength of character to hang on a little longer until the inevitable miracle drug came along. Death, in this secular age, is rarely promoted as an opportunity to pass "through a lowly door to an unimaginable scene," from this veil of tears to the bosom of God.

Juzo Itami, the Japanese filmmaker provides a sharp and poignant commentary:

> Traditionally, when people were about to pass away they stayed at home surrounded by the people close to them. The dying person was the central actor. People had this idea of a gallant death done with deep bravery. People around them accepted the fact that this person is about to pass away and communicated with them. There was a culture of death. People now use science. Science means the defeat of death. They no longer want to look death in the face. Death is worthless, scary, like something you flush from your house. You take this person to the hospital because you don't want this thing to happen in your house.[8]

Is it any surprise that few people can look with equanimity upon their impending death? Is it not much easier — for both patient and bystanders, including the physician — to forge ahead with treatment, any treatment, even useless treatments? To do less would be to admit that one has chosen the wrong path in life, has been singled out by fate to be unworthy of fortunes granted generously to all the others. Anyone who has experienced or sympathized with or imagined such feelings can understand how saying no to medical treatment — any treatment, anything at all — could become a virtually unthinkable option.

Compassion and guilt of bystanders. Almost every doctor who cares for seriously ill patients has had the following experiences: After long and agonizing discussions, members of the family have come to terms with the decision to limit or forgo aggressive, life-prolonging treatments for a loved one and instead emphasize comfort care. Suddenly an estranged relative flies in from a distant state and expresses outrage that the person she has not seen for years is being so cruelly and callously neglected. Or it is a child who lies permanently unconscious after being discovered face down in a backyard swimming pool, the cerebral cortex irrevocably destroyed. The air is filled with cries of blame or guilt. Someone neglected to lock the gate or watch the child closely. The only possible expiation is to keep the unconscious child alive, using every imaginable machine or drug; for as long as the child lives, one can cling to the hope that a miraculous recovery will take place and all will be forgiven. Nor is this phenomenon limited to patients' families. Sometimes physicians who have caused a disastrous outcome, either through bad luck or error, insist on keeping the patient alive despite the utter bleakness of the condition and prognosis. For them, to allow death is to admit failure, or even worse, fault.

However, a compassionate physician will not "do everything" if it is contrary to showing genuine concern for the patient's suffering. Compassion means literally "suffering together with another, participation in suffering" and "when a person is moved by the suffering . . . and by the desire to relieve it."[9] Compassion goes awry when self-deception leads a well-intentioned health professional to think that applying futile treatments will relieve a patient's suffering by achieving a miraculous cure. Alternatively, compassion is ill-informed when a well-meaning doctor or nurse feels that the only way to relieve the patient's suffering or show caring or keep hope alive is by indiscriminately using all possible means at medicine's disposal.

We believe that a compassionate response to a patient's or family's request for futile interventions is open communication, in which the health professional seeks to understand the reasons and motivations for the request. Only then are doctors and nurses well prepared to validate the patient's feelings and explain what medicine can do to relieve suffering. Unfortunately, the impersonal nature of modern medicine has led many health professionals to turn reflexively to high technology fixes (meticulously "following the numbers" of laboratory tests), while underestimating or deriding the importance of low-technology care and ongoing communication. In the modern era, open-ended communication about feelings makes some physicians uncomfortable because it seems inefficient, rather than being directed toward discrete goals. Moreover, whereas technological methods are precise and measurable, conversation in which patients and family members express feelings and fears is open-ended and requires the health professional to relinquish control during the encounter, and perhaps to feel personally sad, disturbed, and vulnerable. To "participate in suffering," as compassion requires, demands health professionals to resist the tendency to deploy futile methods and instead feel emotional pain and turmoil in response to the patient's pain and suffering. The compassionate doctor or nurse thereby acknowledges a common humanity with the patient.

The prospect of a child's death is viewed not only with grief but with a sense of injustice. As just noted, many of us who conduct ethics consultations learn that it is particularly difficult to let a child die. More than the death of an adult, particularly an elderly person, death in a child is seen as premature, cruel, and unjust. As the sociologist Frederic Hafferty showed, physicians-in-training have difficulty accepting the death of younger patients. "[S]tudents" were not only more likely to feel that the terminal status of these [younger] patients was unfair, but that they were also more likely to assume that the patients must feel the same way."[10] In contrast, the students in Hafferty's study were urged in their training to view death in the elderly patient as "something they needed to 'learn from' and 'move beyond'" (194). It should come as no surprise, then, that doctors often feel a greater obligation to continue futile treatments, as though such persistence compensates for fate's unfairness. Why do we respond more emotionally to fatal illness in a child than in an older person? For example, how often does television broadcast appeals by a 50- or 60-year-old seeking an organ transplant, whereas such appeals by children are well known, even legendary? It is as though we do not see an aging person's life as increasing in value with accumulating experience and the development of autonomous values. Rather we seem to picture the lifespan as a limited resource that is consumed, and to regard those who have consumed more life already as deserving less life in the future.

It was not always thus. In ancient Greece and Rome, only adults — indeed, eminent adults, such as rulers and heroes — were considered to have sufficiently deep feelings, capacities for suffering, to be worthy subjects of tragedy. Their misfortunes, therefore, were of great consequence. Children, by contrast, were generally regarded as too innocent and unformed to be capable of great suffering themselves. Their impending deaths evoked profound compassion principally for the adults whose suffering it caused. In the Euripedes play *Medea*, for example, Medea's children are murdered, but the playwright directs the audience's sympathy toward the pain and suffering felt not by these children, but by Jason their father. Imagine a made-for-TV movie today treating children so offhandedly! But regardless of how much our attitudes have changed, no matter how much we treasure or even favor children over adults or elderly people, there still is no reason to pursue futile treatments in *anyone*. Judgments about the benefit or futility of treatments require honest assessments of outcomes in particular patients, not sentimental or stereotypic group comparisons.[11]

In addition to all the factors noted above, there are practical "real world" legal and political reasons why it is difficult to say no to futile treatment.

Fear of lawsuit. Physicians often tell us they fear the legal consequences of forgoing treatment and will even admit their well-known tendency today to practice "defensive medicine." However, as we will discuss in Chapter 6, many physicians have distorted and exaggerated concerns about their legal obligation to continue or offer futile treatments. In our ethics consultations we attempt to deal with legal risks in a measured and realistic way. One potent statement we repeat as often as necessary: No physician has ever suffered a civil judgment or criminal conviction for deliberately (as opposed to negligently) allowing—or even causing—a patient to die. But the fear of facing trial is nevertheless pervasive, and however ill-founded that fear is, physicians often would rather attempt futile treatments than risk being sued.

Fear of adverse media attention. Physicians confronted by angry family members and controversial treatment decisions may consult the hospital attorney. Some hospital attorneys, of course, will properly advise the physician to provide whatever beneficial treatments the patient wants or whatever treatments are in the patient's best interest. But, as these disputes unfold, it often becomes painfully clear that the attorney's client is neither the physician nor the patient but the hospital. Pressured by the attorney and "risk managers," the hospital in turn might pressure the physician to continue inappropriate treatments as a way of avoiding adverse publicity. Thus, public relations are given priority over medical ethics and a genuine and serious application of the law. Families or other parties demanding futile treatments may show they are well aware of this and compound their demands by threatening not only to call their lawyer but also to contact the newspaper and television station.

Money. Families find it easier to demand, and hospitals find it easier to accede to requests for, treatments that are financially painless. An insurance policy that covers continuing treatment on the ventilator for a patient who will never leave the ICU makes continuing such futile treatment much easier for all to justify. Hospitals feel no disinclination to accept reimbursement; and patients and families tend to feel ethically entitled to the futile treatment because it is covered under their insurance plan.

Desperate people deserve anything they want. One of the forces at work when physicians continue to attempt futile treatment is that patients or families make desperate pleas for help. The easiest way to deal with desperate persons is to give them what they want. This force has reached even the highest level of government and become health policy. Activists for diseases such as AIDS and Alzheimer's disease have persuaded the Food and Drug Administration to change its approval policy and to expedite the provision of drugs on a treatment basis before they have been proved to be beneficial. Advocates for the expedited provision of drugs argue that certain conditions are so serious or lethal that patients suffering from these conditions are entitled to any treatments they want—even possibly useless and harmful drugs. Although we sympathize with the desperation motivating these patients and their advocates, we feel a sense of despair as well. Sanctioning dubious drugs before their therapeutic efficacy is established by careful clinical trials only *delays* the discovery of useful drugs. Since only a rare few drugs that initially look promising ultimately turn out to be beneficial, most patients with these conditions will almost certainly experience *more* suffering with their disease as well as with deleterious drug side-effects. Furthermore, many patients will be deceived into thinking that the drugs provided under medical auspices might actually be more beneficial than they really are. And finally, while demanding treatments that may well be futile for themselves, such patients are also depriving future patients of the possibility of swift progress in discovering new treatments.

The well-known ethics and legal scholar George Annas observes that

> the AIDS epidemic has frightened us into believing that medicine will find a cure soon, and this misplaced faith in science has helped erode the distinction between experimentation and therapy; has threatened to transform the United States Food & Drug Administration from a consumer protection agency into a medical technology promotion agency; and has put AIDS patients, already suffering from an incurable disease, at further risk of psychological, physical and financial exploitation by those who would sell them useless drugs. . . . The excuse that patients who are dying with treatment and "have nothing to lose" will not do. Terminally ill patients can be harmed, misused and exploited.[12]

All of the above factors—psychological, cultural, legal, and political—influence medical practice today and must be clearly recognized. Whether or not readers agree with our specific descriptions, they will surely understand the larger implications. If we as a society can find so many reasons not to accept "a kind of striving that is appropriate to a human life,"[13] not to admit to the possibility of futile medical treatment, then physicians will have little incentive to transfer their efforts from aggressive life-saving procedures and seek beneficial and caring alternatives.

CHAPTER 3

WHY WE MUST

SAY NO

Rarely had one of us seen the medical team look so beleaguered. Hunched around the conference room table, the nurses and interns and residents and social worker and attending physician — a bright, well-read, and compassionate woman new to the faculty — all conveyed the same message: We're trapped. The medical record they handed over, only the latest of several volumes, was several inches thick.

Mrs. Boxley (not her real name) was a 92-year-old woman who had been transferred to the hospital from the nursing home because of high fever and suspected pneumonia. It was already the fourth hospitalization this year, which was still several months from being over. Mrs. Moxley had an affliction not uncommon to the elderly, angiodysplasia, a recurrently bleeding malformation of the blood vessels lining her large bowel. Two of the hospital admissions had been for surgical procedures to save her from dying of massive hemorrhage. The other two hospitalizations — like the current one — had been to treat her for episodes of pneumonia resulting from aspiration of food and secretions.

The medical team's gloom was precipitated by circumstances that seemed to be beyond their control, decisions made by the previous team caring for the woman. Those past decisions were forcing them to do things now that made no sense. For example, it was becoming evident that Mrs. Boxley was severely demented, not only when she was sick with pneumonia or recovering from surgery but even when she was as healthy as she could be. Descriptions by her nursing home attendants indicated that, though not unconscious, she seemed to derive no satisfaction or pleasure from her existence. The only sounds she made were grunts and cries of discomfort and pain. Over the last year it had became almost impossible to feed her without causing her to gag and cough and of course to aspirate food into her lungs. Yet whenever a nasogastric feeding tube was laboriously inserted through her nose she cried out even more and kept pulling it out. This time, the nursing home director made clear, she would not take the woman back unless the doctors secured a gastrostomy tube through her abdominal wall directly into her stomach. Because Mrs. Boxley had left no advance directive instructions regarding the treatments she would want under these circumstances and had no relative or friend who could speak on her behalf, the previous medical team had concluded that they had no choice but to comply.

By the time we arrived at the bedside, the feeding gastrostomy tube was in place, the pneumonia was resolving, and the woman was moaning and crying with all her restored strength. Clearly Mrs. Boxley was not deriving any benefit from her treatment. "But what can we do?" the doctors protested. "The decisions already have been made. We're trapped."

As is often the case, the hospital nurses caring for the woman had been the first to demand the ethics consultation. What they were being ordered to do simply made no sense—pumping into her body liquefied nourishment she could not even taste, suctioning her trachea, cleaning up her incontinent wastes, monitoring her vital signs in readiness to leap in with everything from drugs to support her intermittently falling blood pressure to CPR in the event her heart stopped. It violated their most fundamental impulses of compassion, not to mention their professional obligation, to alleviate suffering and provide comfort. At first they aimed their comments angrily at the physicians who had ordered them to carry out the daily tasks. But the physicians threw up their hands. They *agreed* with the nurses. If it had been up to them, they would write a do not attempt resuscitation order and emphasize comfort care. *But what could they do?*

As we went around the conference room table we confirmed to every one's satisfaction that each person there—physician, nurse, social worker—was of the same mind, that because of the patient's condition she was incapable of experiencing any benefit from the treatments aimed at keeping her alive, particularly the gastrostomy tube. In other words, all the health providers caring for Mrs. Boxley considered these treatments futile. All sensed they were participating in something terribly wrong—yet they kept doing it.

What was wrong, we suggested, was that the health providers were failing to recognize that they were not obligated to provide futile treatments. And it was up to them to say no.

How common is this scenario of doctors pursuing treatments they don't believe in? All too common, it seems. Mildred Solomon and her colleagues surveyed 687 physicians and 759 nurses in five different hospitals. Almost half of the providers and almost three-quarters of the doctors admitted that they had acted "against their conscience" in pursuing aggressive treatments on terminally ill patients.[1]

The case of Mrs. Boxley illustrates some of the many reasons why as a matter of professional responsibility these acts should not have happened.

As we emphasized earlier, the goal of medical practice is not to provide any treatment imaginable, but to serve the best interests of the patient by providing *beneficial* treatment. Holding physicians responsible for drawing the line at nonbeneficial, that is, futile, treatment has the effect of demarcating patient rights, but it protects them from abuses as well.

Up to now we have taken the position that treatment decisions offering a benefit should respect patient wishes: Patients are entitled to choose or refuse any such treatments. But in this chapter we will qualify that argument by pointing out that their wishes must be situated in the broader context of family and community needs and interests, not limited to but certainly including practical economic considerations. In other words, sometimes health providers must say no.

THE BORDER BETWEEN PATIENT AUTONOMY AND PHYSICIAN AUTHORITY

Ethicists and a consensus of court decisions up to and including the U.S. Supreme Court *Cruzan* decision have made it clear: Tube and intravenous feeding and hydration are to be regarded as medical treatments which, like any other medical treatments, can be stopped under appropriate circumstances. As the ethics consultant in Mrs. Boxley's case, we recommended that, of course, if she had any relatives or friends involved in her care, the doctors should try their best to get them to understand that the tube feeding was providing no therapeutic benefit. For their own peace of mind, it would be preferable for them to accept and be part of the decision to withdraw it. But ultimately it was up to the doctors to say no.

The doctors listened and agreed, but it soon became apparent they still were not happy. The tube was already in place. We might have been able to say no *before* it was inserted, but we can't just pull it out *now* . . . can we?

The answer, we said, is yes — once again, if the treatment is not benefiting the patient. Withholding and withdrawing futile treatments are regarded in the law as equivalent acts. If the treatment is not indicated, that is all that matters — stopping is the same as not starting. Discontinuing tube feeding, or "pulling the plug" on a mechanical ventilator, for example, is no different from discontinuing any inappropriate medical treatment. Nor does it matter whether the treatment is hand-delivered out of a bottle of pills, squirted through a syringe, or propelled by electrical power. As expressed in the influential California Appellate Court decision, *Barber v. Los Angeles County Superior Court,*

> each pulsation of the respirator or each drop of fluid introduced into the patient's body by intravenous feeding devices is comparable to a manually administered injection or item of medication. Hence, "disconnecting" of the mechanical devices is comparable to the withholding the manually administered injection or medication.[2]

The *Barber* decision had been announced in 1983, almost ten years before the medical team brought their plight to the medical ethicist. Since then it has been cited innumerable times in high courts around the country as one of many precedents for withdrawing unwanted and futile treatments. Similar position statements have been issued by the American Medical Association (1986), the American Nurses' Association (1988), the American Academy of Neurology (1989), and the American Thoracic Society (1991). Yet even for sophisticated physicians in an academic medical center, it was as though these events had never happened. As we have already seen and will see again in this book, medical treatments continue to be imposed and demanded in ways that defy common sense.

As Solomon and her colleagues observed to their chagrin, most of the 687 physicians she interviewed

> were uncertain about what the law, ethics, and their respective professional standards say on this matter [withdrawing treatment]. In addition to this uncertainty, the interviewed respondents reported being

less likely to withdraw treatments than to withhold them for a variety of other reasons, including psychological discomfort with actively stopping a life-sustaining intervention; discomfort with the public nature of the act, which might occasion a lawsuit from disapproving witnesses even if the decision were legally correct; and fear of sanction by peer review boards.[3]

We have already seen how health care providers, courts and politicians lacking a true understanding of the obligations of the medical profession and its limits as well as its powers, ran roughshod over the reasonable demands of the Cruzan parents to free their daughter from being maintained in a state of perpetual unconsciousness by the medical treatment. In Chapter 6 we will see that in some court cases, the pressure for futile treatment came from the other side, the family. In one situation, the husband of Helga Wanglie persuaded the court to compel doctors against their judgment to continue life support on his wife, who had been irrevocably unconscious, in a permanent vegetative state, for over a year. In another case, the mother of Baby K demanded that repeated emergency life-saving treatment be carried out on her daughter, who was born without most of her brain, a condition known as anencephaly.

In all such instances, medicine was viewed as a force to be exercised on demand rather than judiciously and selectively directed at illness. Unfortunately we are beginning to see the consequences of this view. For although the powers of modern medicine have inspired awe, it is becoming increasingly apparent they also arouse a contrary view in the mind of the public, an inordinate fear of being trapped in a modern, dehumanizing technology with no hope of escape.

One startling bit of evidence for the pervasiveness of this latter view is the popularity of a do-it-yourself suicide book published by the Hemlock Society, an advocacy group supporting voluntary euthanasia.[4] Astonishingly, the book was a bestseller and grist for widespread pontification. What could possibly be so appealing about an instruction manual for taking one's life?

The answer seems to reflect a deep distrust felt by many individuals toward physicians. Patients worry: Will my doctors make humane and compassionate end-of-life decisions? Or will they ignore suffering and force on me unwanted technological indignities? These people—and they seem to number in the many thousands—are apparently drawn to the idea of taking their lives (and their deaths) into their own hands. In other words, as a result of Nancy Cruzan and other highly visible cases, medical treatment has come to be viewed by many as an unleashed menace rather than as a beneficent healing process.

Blame for this state of affairs is passed out freely. Some point to physicians and the entire "medical-industrial complex" which, for venal or misguided moral reasons, insist upon perpetuating life-preserving treatments to absurd extremes. Others find fault with patients and families, who while striving for miracles or heroic actions, demand unrelentingly that "everything be done." The fact is, our pluralistic society—through courts and legislatures—has not articulated a coherent set of values to effectively counter extremes from either side.

Although most higher courts have supported the right to refuse unwanted treatments—even forcing hospitals to assume the costs of such treatments when pursued—they have not been reassuringly consistent. In one egregious case, a high New York State court forced an elderly woman's family to pay tens of thousand of dollars for hospital treatment that provided no benefit to the patient and which the patient expressly did not want.[5]

The unpredictability of the legal aspect, agonizing as it is to patients and families, should not be surprising. Lawyers, and consequently judges, rigorously trained in civil and criminal matters, have concentrated on malpractice and liability rather than on ethical issues. Sometimes their ignorance about basic biology and medicine, critical to rendering sound and reasoned judgments, is appalling.

Nor can we expect state and federal legislation (again, for the most part, the work of lawyers) to provide more than the most clumsy guidelines. Medical treatments represent an ever-changing kaleidoscope of art and science and human relationships. Decisions at the bedside are complicated enough without bringing in "roving strangers" with their own narrow and exclusive moral agendas attached to voting blocks, whose activities almost guarantee that legislative advances in medical ethics decision-making will be limited and perverse, if they take place at all.

Given all these confounding obstacles, is there any possibility that the medical profession and the public will recognize the necessity to forgo futile treatments? Surprisingly, we are optimistic. As we discuss in Chapters 8 and 9, much of what we describe here has already ignited a debate among physicians about medical futility. It is our hope that this book will bring attention to the subject and foster critical discussion among not only members of the health care and legal professions but also society at large.

MONEY

One obvious reason why society must begin to resist inappropriate and nonbeneficial medical treatment is that it can no longer afford to waste valuable resources. As George Lundberg, editor of the *Journal of the American Medical Association,* stated in a recent editorial: "We Americans value health, and we don't mind spending a lot of money for it. But we want value for our money, and we are currently convinced that, as a nation, we are not getting our money's worth. This must change."[6]

Dire warnings of spiraling health-care costs are reported almost daily in the media. Already our country spends about 14 percent of its gross domestic product on health care, almost double the percentage spent in Great Britain and well above every other civilized country in Europe and Canada. Further, those countries provide insurance coverage for everyone, whereas in the U.S. an estimated thirty-five to forty million people live every day threatened by the prospect of illness without adequate health insurance.

Not only are health-care expenditures already high, they are increasing at a rate of 12–15 percent a year, about four to five times the rate of economic growth. The United States Commerce Department estimates that in 1994 health-care spending will easily exceed $1 trillion. Many factors contribute to the rising cost of health care: the proliferation of expensive, high-technology medical equipment; the aging of the population; and the increasing use of costly treatments for illnesses such as cancer, AIDS, and heart disease.

Unless we are willing to reduce the amount of money devoted to other important priorities such as education, roads, transportation, communication, and so forth, we as a nation are going to have to make a first-order decision, namely, to decrease the overall expenditure on health care. President Clinton stated this forcefully when he presented the outlines of his new health plan to the National Governors' Association in 1993: "If health care costs had been held in check — that is, to inflation plus growth — since 1980, state and local governments would have an average of 75 percent more funding for public school budgets. In 1993, . . . states spent more on Medicaid than on higher education for the first time."[7]

While making first-order choices, we will also have to make some second-order decisions, namely, choosing areas of health care to reduce, thereby saving resources for other areas of health care. However, as we have indicated in the previous chapter and will discuss in Chapter 5, it is not enough to view the problem merely as cost-containment and rationing. Making choices on these grounds will be time-consuming and difficult for society. But as we wait for the process to go forth, are we really willing to forsake other vital needs in order to pursue futile treatments? As we have pointed out, if certain treatments offer no reasonable chance of providing a benefit, they simply should not be attempted.

If some fourteen thousand to thirty-five thousand patients in permanent vegetative state are being kept alive at a cost that is estimated to be somewhere between $1 billion and $7 billion per year, this futile medical treatment is not a rationing or cost containment issue, but rather a misuse of medicine itself.

On the other hand, if there are about fifteen hundred potential donor hearts that could be used for transplantation each year and some three to four thousand patients with failing hearts who would benefit by a heart transplant (about a third of whom die while waiting), this is not a question of futile medical treatment but rather a difficult problem in making choices. The choice may be one of cost containment (i.e., perhaps on the whole we would rather limit the number of heart transplants to ten thousand a year and use the money saved for other worthy treatments). Or it could be a rationing problem in that we decide to make use of all fifteen thousand donor hearts (and more if available) but allocate them according to some criteria that may combine medical as well as social characteristics. But it is important that we not complicate the issue unnecessarily by spending money and resources uselessly on futile treatments.

These should be eliminated from the ledger of obligations to maximize the availability of treatments that do work.

How does all this apply to Mrs. Boxley? It is perhaps fruitful to contrast our view with that of the ethicist Daniel Callahan. In his book *Setting Limits,* Callahan proposes that "after a person has lived out a natural life span [which would "normally be expected by the late 70s or early 80s,"] medical care should no longer be oriented to resisting death."[8] Thus, by his criterion, the 92-year old Mrs. Boxley would no longer be eligible for life-saving medical technologies. But what would Callahan do about her feeding tube? Apparently he would continue to use it to keep her alive because he is opposed to withdrawing artificial nutrition and hydration. Following Callahan's set of contrary rules, Mrs. Boxley would end up being kept in her state of unalleviated suffering and dementia until taken away by a cardiac arrest or other dramatic event requiring a more obvious employment of medical technology. Such an approach strikes us as lacking a coherent purpose, namely the benefit of the patient.

We analyze Mrs. Boxley's case differently. First of all, it does not matter how old she is. She could be 20, 30, 40, any age up to and beyond her nineties, she would still not be a candidate for any medical treatment that provided no benefit. Sedation, pain medication, bathing, moistening of the lips—clearly, these would benefit her, since she is suffering. Oxygen and antibiotics might also be of help if they alleviated the distress of her pneumonia. All these treatments are aimed at symptoms we believe she is capable of experiencing. But the feeding tube serves no purpose other than keeping her alive to endure more suffering. Therefore, it is futile and should be stopped and replaced by measures undertaken to their maximum powers that provide comfort and dignity.

MISUSE OF TECHNOLOGY

At the pioneering Seattle Artificial Kidney Center early in the 1960s, patients dying of kidney disease were selected for the newly minted life-saving dialysis treatment by an ethics committee that reviewed criteria including age, gender, marital status, number of dependents, net worth, educational background, occupation, past performance, and future potential. Even letters of recommendation were solicited. This process was adopted by other medical centers around the country. In short time the anguish experienced by such committees, not to mention that experienced by candidates undergoing the selection process (the majority of whom were necessarily rejected), put pressure on Congress to enact the Medicare End Stage Renal Disease Program in 1972. This amendment provided universal access to treatment at no cost to the patient and under no prescribed limitations. Experts at the time predicted that enrollment in the program would level off by 1992 to ninety thousand patients. How did their predictions turn out? By 1992 almost twice that number of Medicare patients with end-stage renal disease had entered treatment, and the growth in enrollment shows no sign of leveling off. For as soon as financial barriers were removed, renal dialysis and transplantation began to be offered to patients with conditions that had never been envisioned by the original proponents: patients with severe diabetes, heart disease, liver disease, and even those in permanent vegetative state started receiving regular and frequent renal dialysis. Now the annual per patient cost for the End Stage Renal Disease Program is nine times higher than for other Medicare patients, and a program that once was predicted to cost about $1 billion a year at most now costs more than $7 billion per year. As one writer commented in the *New England Journal of Medicine:* "The End Stage Renal Disease Program demonstrates the humane impulse that strikes Americans periodically to act on behalf of a vulnerable population. The legislative history of the program suggests that this impulse is driven more by emotions, timing, and the political need to expand benefits than by rational planning."[9]

Intensive care units (ICUs) were developed in the late 1960s to provide a temporary high-technology environment to enable teams of medical providers to rescue patients with acute, serious, life-threatening disease. Patients were expected either to survive and be transferred out of the unit or to die. All this has changed. Today, in our ethics consultations we often discuss patients who have been in the ICU for many months. We even have been asked to consult on patients who have inhabited the ICU for more than a year, with no realistic chance of leaving until they die.

Cardiopulmonary resuscitation (CPR) was developed in the 1960s as a rapid emergency procedure to rescue patients with acute life-threatening cardiac arrest. These patients were expected to survive and resume their usual life outside the hospital. Today CPR is applied on vast numbers of patients who have little chance of surviving even to hospital discharge. Such patients may have terminal cancer or advanced and debilitating failure in several organ systems—lungs, kidneys, heart, liver, bone marrow, and blood—that need continuing support, substitution or replenishment. In the past their cardiac arrest, which today is so frantically attacked, would have been considered a welcome event, a "good death," putting a merciful end to their life.

The above examples are illustrations of how superbly effective advances in medical treatments have become purposeless rituals without reasonable goals. In all of these cases, the intervention was viewed by those first employing it in a far more limited and directed way than has subsequently evolved. One can argue, of course, that there could be many good reasons to expand the applications of an effective technology beyond its original intentions. However, the expansive use of these technologies has often gone unabated and unexamined or simplistically justified on the "life-is-priceless" principle.

An example of this attitude is reflected in the announcement to the press by the chief surgeon at Children's Hospital of Philadelphia after a highly publicized separation of Siamese twin girls, which offered one infant an exceedingly slim chance of long-term survival at an estimated total cost of care at over $1 million: "There has been a unanimous consensus that if it is possible to save one life, then it is worth doing this." (The child died a year later, never having left the hospital, never having been weaned from a ventilator.) Professor Ronald Dworkin, a scholar of ethics and law responded: "We must face the fact that this is an impossible, even absurd, ideal."[10] A senior vice president of therapeutics, justifying her pharmaceutical company's $20,000 to $60,000 charge per year for treating a single patient with a single drug, stated: "If there's a scientific way of treating a disease, we have to develop it, and we as a nation have to figure out how to pay for it."[11]

Only now is this "unanimous consensus" and "damn-the-torpedoes" attitude being challenged and replaced by calls for research to examine not only the cost but also the effectiveness of treatments in certain clinical circumstances. Already this challenge is bearing fruit with regard to uncovering futile treatments. For example, Dr. Kathy Faber-Langendoen and her colleagues, after reviewing the thirteen-year experience of patients who required mechanical ventilation at the highly regarded University of Minnesota Bone Marrow Transplant Program, called upon physicians to note how abysmal their results had been.[12] Of the 191 patients who had to be put on the ventilator only 6 (3 percent) were alive six months later. None of the patients who required mechanical ventilation within 90 days of the transplant lived more than 100 days, and none of the patients over 40 years of age lived more than a month. And so, after thirteen years of employing this invasive treatment, the researchers concluded that mechanical ventilation "is rarely effective in achieving long-term survival in adult BMT [bone marrow transplant] recipients, especially older patients and those early in their transplant course." Which means that during all those years, many bone marrow transplant patients were forced to endure the additional pain and suffering and indignity of a treatment that resulted in no survival outside the hospital, because physicians had never systematically asked the relevant question, Does it work or is it futile?, before automatically hooking the patient up to the machine.

Stephen C. Schoenbaum, a Harvard physician, expressed dismay at the failure of physicians to examine their "bias toward action."[13] Faber-Langendoen encountered it, and it propelled the surgeons who inserted Mrs. Boxley's feeding tube.

THE GLARE OF AUTONOMY

We have already referred to the evolution of the doctor-patient relationship from one that allowed what is now considered excessive paternalism to one that places great emphasis on patient autonomy. This evolution can almost be regarded as a paradigm shift, to adopt an expression used to describe the abrupt changes in the ways scientists historically have viewed the physical world.[14] In the early 1960s, when a group of internists practicing in the United States were asked whether they would inform their patients that they had a grave form of cancer, as many as 90 percent of the physicians expressed reluctance and uncertainty about telling the truth to their patients.[15] A few years later, a similar survey showed exactly the opposite: 90 percent of American physicians studied said they certainly *would* tell the patient the truth.[16] During this period of time—coinciding with the dramatic and much-celebrated social upheavals of the sixties—a remarkable transformation took place in medical teaching and practice.

One of the authors is witness to this vivid change. When he was a medical student in the mid-1950s, a senior physician, who was revered for his compassionate care of patients, gave this advice to all the physicians-in-training after examining on rounds a woman in the last stages of cancer. The frightened woman had asked him directly if she was going to die of her cancer, and he replied kindly, but evasively, "We're all going to die." Later, away from the woman, he counseled us: "Do not tell *her* she has incurable cancer. But make sure someone in the family knows the truth." At the time it was considered the height of clinical wisdom.[17] Today, in the United States, it would be regarded as unthinkable as well as unethical, and even in most cases illegal, not to answer the patient kindly but honestly.

This strong emphasis on "patients' rights" is now a salient and valuable quality in medical decision-making. However, just as physicians abused their kindness in attempting to withhold the truth in the past, sometimes patients abuse the power inherent in their right to make choices about their medical care. Some patients have interpreted their right to control what is done to them by physicians as a right to demand anything they want from physicians. In asserting this right they have created a kind of "glare of autonomy," blinding participants to all other considerations while converting all their desires and dreams into a medical context.

In the case of Mrs. Boxley, the glare of autonomy was even more powerful. In the *absence* of permission from her or from someone empowered to speak on her behalf, the physicians felt blocked from pursuing a course of treatment and care everyone agreed was the most appropriate and humane.

EXHAUSTING THE COMMONS

During medieval and preindustrial times, a central green provided a place for English and other European peasants and yeomen to graze their animals. The commons was a communal resource for the benefit of all, and a sense of restraint controlled each family's use of the green. Obviously, if one commoner decided to take advantage of the grazing privilege by adding an extra cow or two, the effect would hardly be noticed. But what if all the neighbors picked up the idea? What if they all increased the number of cows they set out to graze? Eventually all would suffer because the commons would be exhausted. Instead, by mutual consent, they all resisted the temptation to increase their own advantage at the expense of the community at large. Today we often neglect the notion of the commons in our current emphasis on autonomy and individualism. But the concept is relevant to medical resources.[18] The fact is a kind of medical commons exists for all patients. It is not made up merely of material things—institutional space, equipment, supplies and personnel—but it consists also of the psyche of care-givers, both loved ones and professionals. These too can become depleted, worn out, exhausted.

In the case of Mrs. Boxley, we could see the beginning of serious burnout problems that frequently occur among health providers in high-intensity settings, particularly when they feel they are pursuing measures that have no point. All health-care providers—doctors, nurses, social workers—are motivated and trained and expected to devote their best efforts to either curing or caring for the patients under their responsibility. Every day their efforts are subjected to great physical and emotional pressures. We could sense the wearing down such dedicated, compassionate people feel when they see their efforts consumed and distorted by fruitless demands. And we knew that inevitably, this exhaustion of the commons would affect other patients under their care.

We have also seen an exhaustion of the commons occurring among family members responsible for the care of severely handicapped children or severely debilitated adults and elderly individuals.[19] Families will make remarkable sacrifices, rallying to the assistance of one member, as long as the burdens are proportionate to the anticipated outcomes and the benefits to the patient are evident. At times, however, we have seen health providers impose on their own colleagues and on family members an unrealistic patient-centered ethic that fails to recognize the community in which we all draw sustenance. Just as the individual should be respected and valued, so should the community. And so, at times we must say no to futile treatment for no other reason than to prevent the destructive consequences extending to others who are inescapably affected by the treatment of the patient.

BALANCING THE CLAIMS OF SINGLE-ISSUE ADVOCATES

Nowhere is the balancing of individual needs versus community needs more explicit than in the conflicts that are generated by single-issue advocates. As described in Chapter 1, the Cruzan family members were subjected to the aggressive protests of "pro-life" groups seeking to overturn the family's hard-won decision to terminate Nancy Cruzan's treatment. Many such groups have agendas that arise from belief systems they wish to impose on society in general and on the medical profession in particular. During the Reagan and Bush era, such groups were able to impose a "gag rule" on publicly funded clinics that provided family planning services including abortion counseling and referral. Many of these advocacy groups hold a vitalist view of life, condemning any abatement of treatment as long as some biological state, including permanent unconsciousness, continues. Or, in viewing permanent unconsciousness as another variant of mental disability, they trivialize the needs of patients who really *are* disabled and distract attention from those who really *could* benefit from more resources directed at their needs.

What would these "roving strangers" have done had they been aware of the ethics conference devoted to Mrs. Boxley? It is too easy to imagine a media campaign that ignores the complexity of balancing benefits and burdens by simplistically protesting the horrendous "killing of a poor lonely old woman." Thus, before courts and legislatures bend to such relentless proselytizing, it is important for an enlightened society to make these issues public, to examine them openly and critically. Ultimately, we hope, thoughtful standards will be fashioned that are compatible with both the values of society and the true ends of the medical profession.

CURBING INAPPROPRIATE AND COVERT ABUSES

In our ethics consultations we have identified a variety of factors that influence medical treatments. These factors can lead physicians both to curtail and to continue treatments inappropriately. Is the patient old, the disease unattractive, the treatment complicated? Health care providers sometimes find ways to limit their efforts because there are no clear measures by which to judge them. Is the patient wealthy, important, perhaps even a member of the medical profession? Then no amount of treatment is regarded as too expensive or futile. Does the patient have HIV infection? Physicians are notoriously reluctant to expose themselves to the risk of infection no matter how slight. Once again, there are no standards by which to judge the activities of the health care providers. And without some clear set of standards, physicians and patients have no way to examine critically the underlying justification for medical decisions. Thus, we must say no to futile medical treatment as a way of clarifying those treatments that are not futile, those that are obligatory, and those that lie within the realm of patient choice. These steps will serve not only to protect a medical profession fearful of liability but also to safeguard the interests of patients like Mrs. Boxley.

CHAPTER 4

FAMILIES

WHO WANT

EVERYTHING

DONE

Helga Wanglie was 85 years old when she suffered an accident common to all of us, but potentially deadly for the elderly: she tripped on a rug. She tumbled to the floor and broke her hip. During the time it takes for the fracture to heal, patients confined to bed such as Mrs. Wanglie can fall prey to blood clots, bed sores, and pneumonia. Up to 20 percent of elderly patients with broken hips die, and many of the survivors never walk again.[1] Many people, though, probably would consider Mrs. Wanglie's outcome—the irreversible unconsciousness of permanent vegetative state—the worst outcome of all.[2]

During her hospitalization at Hennepin County Medical Center, in Minneapolis, Mrs. Wanglie developed respiratory failure requiring emergency tracheal intubation and placement on a mechanical respirator. Despite months of intensive efforts by doctors and technicians, she was never again able to breathe on her own. During these months Mrs. Wanglie remained conscious and aware of her surroundings. She was able to communicate with visiting family members, and she was able to acknowledge when she was in pain or uncomfortable. Yet when asked about her future treatment wishes, she gave ambiguous and inconsistent answers.

She was transferred to a medical facility that specializes in the care of respirator-dependent patients. There she suffered a cardiac arrest. Although resuscitated and rushed by ambulance to a nearby acute-care hospital, she never regained consciousness. Faced with clinical signs portending that her unconsciousness would be permanent, a physician asked the patient's husband, son, and daughter to consider withdrawing life-support measures, such as the mechanical respirator. But they refused. Instead, the family arranged to have Mrs. Wanglie moved back to Hennepin County Medical Center. There, after observing her for several weeks, the doctors informed the family of their concurrence that Mrs. Wanglie was in permanent vegetative state and would never recover. They, too, recommended that life-sustaining treatment be withdrawn since it was not benefiting her. But the Wanglie family responded that doctors should not play God, that even suggesting such a step showed moral decay in our civilization, since a miracle could occur.[3]

It was never clear to the physicians whether the family's demands to continue life-support represented Mrs. Wanglie's specific wishes or their own. When asked early in his wife's illness, Mr. Wanglie told the medical team that his wife had never discussed her views on life-sustaining treatment; yet later he asserted: "My wife always stated to me that if anything happened to her so that she could not take care of herself, she didn't want anything done to shorten or prematurely take her life." He claimed to base this view on their religious and personal beliefs. "Only God can take life," he stated, "and the doctors should not play God."[4]

Over the next several months, the medical team followed the wishes of the patient's family to continue aggressive medical treatment. Mrs. Wanglie was kept on the mechanical ventilator and tube feedings. She was vigorously treated with airway suctioning and antibiotics for recurring pneumonia. Blood tests were performed frequently to facilitate correction of any chemical or fluid imbalances. But because of the irrevocable destruction of her cerebral cortex (demonstrable by CAT scan) and her multiple medical complications, the medical staff caring for Mrs. Wanglie remained convinced that recovery was impossible and, therefore, her life-sustaining ventilator should be discontinued.

At this point, the notion of medical futility should, in our view, have been directly addressed and presented openly for society's enlightenment and consideration. The chance of restoring Mrs. Wanglie to any semblance of consciousness was nil. Were the physicians *obligated* to keep alive a permanently unconscious patient, whose brain was irrevocably destroyed, because the family remained hopeful that "a miracle could occur"? Or were the physicians free to act—to withdraw or continue Mrs. Wanglie's life-sustaining ventilator—guided only by their conscience? Or were they not completely free to make the choice without considering existing guidelines of the profession, but also not compelled to follow them? Or were physicians, as a matter of professional ethics, *obligated not to provide futile treatments*? We will explore these questions in greater detail in Chapter 7.

Interestingly, the hospital's medical director tried to add institutional support to the physicians' assertion of professional ethics in withdrawing life-sustaining treatment on the grounds of medical futility: "All medical consultants agree with [the attending physician's] conclusion that continued use of mechanical ventilation and other forms of life-sustaining treatment are no longer serving the patient's personal medical interest. We do not believe that the hospital is obliged to provide inappropriate medical treatment that cannot advance a patient's personal interest."[5]

Why then didn't the health care providers live up to their declared responsibility of withholding "inappropriate medical treatment"? Sadly, the medical center authorities bypassed the physicians and instead consulted their general legal counsel, who chose not to test the issues of medical futility. Rather than following the wishes of the physicians to bring to court the substantive matter—Was Mrs. Wanglie's ventilator futile and were the physicians obligated to provide it?—the Hennepin County Medical Center lawyers chose to engage in a tactical battle with the Wanglie family, a decision that shaped the future course of events.

First, they asked Mr. Wanglie, an attorney himself, to transfer his wife to another hospital more sympathetic with his views, but he refused. The medical center then proposed that if Mr. Wanglie insisted on continuing treatments the physicians regarded as inappropriate, he obtain a court order. Again he refused. The medical center then decided to go to court to remove Mr. Wanglie's decision-making authority.

An interesting sidelight is worth noting. The physicians wanted to test this issue on a patient in whom neither the hospital nor the county had a financial stake in terminating treatment in order to avoid any suggestion of conflict of interest. In fact, they avoided seeking court permission to withdraw treatment on another patient who happened to be in the hospital at the same time in a similar condition—but who happened to be on welfare. They reasoned that if the doctors were seen by the media as trying to terminate treatment on a welfare patient, how could they avoid "bad headlines" charging that they were trying to kill patients to save money?

But Mrs. Wanglie's hospital treatment presented no such difficulty. All her costs—approximately $800,000 by the time she died—

were fully reimbursed by Medicare and a private supplementary insurance plan. Thus, no one could reasonably claim that the hospital was opposed to Mrs. Wanglie's treatment on grounds of self-interest. In fact (a little known and generally unreported fact), the Wanglie family had a financial interest in keeping the patient in the hospital. Neither Medicare nor their supplementary insurance policy would have covered Mrs. Wanglie's costs if she were in a nursing home. Medicaid welfare would have covered her nursing-home care, but only after she had spent down her assets, including the pension she had hoped to leave to her family. Unfortunately, this is not an unusual experience. Whatever devotion family members might feel for a loved one, their demands for aggressive life-sustaining treatments often cannot avoid being influenced by budgetary matters. Prolonging or curtailing life can have significant consequences on survivors, ranging from the loss of life savings to the termination of monthy disability checks.

In any event, the hospital decided to try to remove Mr. Wanglie from the case. The medical center lawyers asked the court to appoint an independent conservator for Mrs. Wanglie to decide whether the mechanical ventilator keeping her alive was benefiting her. They then hoped for a second hearing on whether the hospital was obligated to continue the ventilator if it was deemed nonbeneficial. But Mr. Wanglie intercepted this two-stage strategy by immediately cross-filing, requesting that *he* be appointed his wife's conservator. The court understandably granted his request. Who, the court reasoned, could better represent Helga Wanglie's views and interests than her own husband?

And so a major opportunity to bring the issue of medical futility to the attention of the courts and to the attention of the public was lost in the smoke of legal pot-shots.

As this case illustrates, the forces leading to the pursuit of futile medical treatment are not limited to the medical profession or to intruding outsiders. Sometimes they come from families who want "everything done." In fact, according to Dr. Edwin H. Cassem, Chief of Psychiatry and head of the Optimum Care Committee at the Massachusetts General Hospital, something akin to the Wanglie scenario has been the most common to trigger an ethics consultation in that committee's twenty-year experience: families insisting that the patient be given treatments physicians regard as futile.[6]

And so, in this chapter we address the questions: Why do families and loved ones make such demands, pleading for treatments that are against all reason? How should physicians and other health professionals respond to such demands?

WHY DO FAMILIES AND LOVED ONES WANT "EVERYTHING DONE"?

In a personal anecdote, the medical ethicist Norman Daniels provided insight into the universality of the Wanglie phenomenon: the conflicted emotional state that assails families who want "everything done," including medical treatments that have been prolonged beyond the point of usefulness. He recounted how his aged great-aunt became seriously ill and was rushed to an intensive-care hospital, where exhaustive efforts were made to extend her life. The woman's daughter (Professor Daniels's cousin) sought to reassure him: "The doctors are doing everything to save her." But when Daniels suggested that "perhaps it was time to let her die peacefully," he was rebuked. "It's my mother—I can't do that," the woman responded. Daniels then asked her whether she would want her own daughter to treat her some day the way she was treating her mother. "God forbid," the daughter exclaimed. "When my time comes, I just want to go."[7]

The striking feature about this exchange is how it exposes the contrast between what we want for ourselves and what we demand, or feel obligated to provide, for those we love. Is this why Mr. Wanglie found it so difficult to agree to stop medical treatments that were doing his wife no good? Did the decision uncover deep feelings of guilt or animosity in relation to his wife? Did he perceive the life-extending treatments to be a way of proving his "undying" love, demanding them in order to meet his obligation as a good and faithful husband? Was the idea of allowing Mrs. Wanglie to die tainted by a sense that withdrawing life-prolonging treatment would signify that she was unworthy of respect and dignity? Had the treatments become transformed into a symbolic ritual? Had they been diverted into a means of benefitting Mr. Wanglie rather than his wife, a way of postponing his own inevitable loss?

Daniels's story reveals how our love for another person can

cause us to demand more for that person than we would demand (or even permit) for ourselves. Boundless love suggests that there can be no limits to what we owe to the object of our love. Yet, making extraordinary (and useless) efforts as an expression of love has an empty ring to it when those efforts do not benefit the object of love. If Mr. Wanglie were intent on proving his love for his wife, he chose ways that did not benefit *her.* She was beyond all comprehension. We can understand the depth of his feelings; but must we require that the doctors, nurses, and other health-care providers, indeed society at large, participate in gestures that do not serve the best interests of *the patient,* his wife?

It is helpful to contrast our demands for loved ones not only with our desires for ourselves but also with our perceived obligations to other people — strangers. Philosophers have observed that we tend to feel we owe more to those with whom we are intimate than we owe to complete strangers. The *special* obligations that flow from personal relationships are not only stronger in *degree* but different in *kind.* Friends and family members may feel an unlimited obligation to provide nurturing, personal time, life savings, even life itself. Indeed, lovers sometimes do take their own lives, rather than be without their loved ones — though this serves no useful purpose to the loved one. What has happened, of course, is that the person one loves may have become such a central part of a person's life that the loss of that person is tantamount to losing one's *self.* Perhaps underneath Mr. Wanglie's demands for continued treatment was the question he could not face: If I am no longer her husband, who am I?

And so, regardless of whether we owe unlimited expressions of love to spouses and siblings and children and parents, it is not surprising that we *feel* that we do. Ordinarily, going out of our way to help those we love strengthens and reinforces the bonds of our relationships. In the medical setting, however, when treatment has become futile, "doing everything" can become a cruel parody. It is not that the impulse to do everything possible is itself is wrongheaded; rather we need to rethink what it means to do our utmost when a loved one is hopelessly ill and dying. In Mrs. Wanglie's case, for example, Mr. Wanglie would have done the utmost for his wife by allowing her to die with as much kindness and dignity as possible, free of useless life-sustaining machinery. Rather than unthinkingly following Mr. Wanglie's demands, the health-care providers would have better lived up to their professional obligations to Mrs. Wanglie by supporting actions that, when the alternatives are futile, allowed her to become part of a cherished past as a beloved person rather than as a permanent vegetative "state."

HOW SHOULD PHYSICIANS RESPOND TO DEMANDS FOR FUTILE TREATMENT?

John Paris, a priest, and Frank E. Reardon, a philosopher, issue the challenge very bluntly: "How do we respond to families and physicians who seek refuge from unwanted painful reality in 'futile end-stage gestures'?"[8]

Some find the answer all too easy: Patients and families are entitled to full decision-making authority, including even irrational choices, as protection against "the medical profession's intent and power to maintain its paternalistic authority,"[9] according to Troy A. Brennan.

But Paris and Reardon have little patience with that notion:

> With an approach that places near control in the hands of the patient, no moral legitimacy is given to a physician's refusal of requested treatment. The physician is reduced from moral agent — one with professional responsibilities and limits on what may legitimately be done — and transformed into an extension of the patients' (or families') whim, fantasy or unrealizable hopes and desires. Such a relationship not only distorts the physician's role, it destroys the very autonomy it was designed to enhance.[10]

We agree. Do we really want physicians to be forced to include "whim, fantasy, or unrealizable hopes and desires" in their therapeutic armamentarium? Without "at least a modicum of potential benefit, as seen from the medical perspective," ethicists Allan Brett and Laurence B. McCullough argue, "the whole raison d'être of the physician-patient interaction disappears."[11]

"DON'T LET THEM GIVE UP ON ME"

Sometimes, of course, it seems easier to submit to unreasonable demands than to challenge them. But what are patients (or more often their families) really asking from physicians?[12]

In a poignant letter to the editor of the *New York Times,* Janet Rivkin Zuckerman suggests that physicians who unquestioningly pursue futile treatments either out of misguided duty or in response to families' demands demonstrate a distressing poverty of imagination: "Isn't it possible that if physicians were more highly developed and educated in doctor-patient relations — that is, in empathy, understanding and communication — it would offset their driving need always to *do* something?"[13]

In other words, it struck Ms. Zuckerman that in looking for empathy, understanding, and communication, patients and families want physicians not to become reflexive automatons. Yes, patients and families want their physicians to be skillful and knowledgeable masters of the science and technology of medicine. But they also want their physicians to be wise counselors whose understanding embraces not only their patients but also the human condition.

We believe that underlying many of the demands to "do everything" is the fear of abandonment. Does the doctor consider me (or my father) no longer worthy of her attention? There are many indirect ways these fears may be expressed by the patient or by the patient's loved ones. For example, Robert M. Veatch and Carol Mason Spicer, two Kennedy Institute ethicists, describe a 36-year-old man admitted to the hospital with symptoms of advanced AIDS:

> He was placed on a ventilator and became mentally incompetent. The clinicians concluded that further aggressive care would be futile, but the patient's lover intervened, saying that he and the patient had discussed these matters openly and that the patient had asked that everything be done. He was quoted as saying, "Don't let them give up on me."[14]

Veatch and Spicer draw the conclusion from this heart-rending plea that by "everything" the patient meant all the *life-saving* procedures in the medical arsenal, including presumably CPR, mechanical ventilation, renal dialysis, major surgery, or whatever else might conceivably be of use to keep the man's body alive.

But we regard this as a simplistic interpretation of what medicine has to offer the dying patient, and we draw a far different conclusion. To us the patient's cry poignantly reveals what has become lost in medical practice and what is missing in the futility debate. If medical decision-making at the end of life is nothing more than deciding whether or not to "pull the plug" or "pound on the chest," a patient who is not offered life-saving treatment might reasonably wonder: Do the doctors deem me unworthy of their attention and concern? Am I no longer of value? Am I being discarded? Understandably the patient or the patient's loved ones might respond with a desperate plea to "do everything," meaning do everything that gives dignity and respect to the remaining moments of life.

The futility debate then degenerates into a conflict between physician and patient (or surrogate or family member) over who decides if a particular life-saving treatment is futile and should not be attempted. Those who argue on behalf of physician-determined futility will emphasize the limits of the medical profession's obligations to provide inappropriate treatments. In rebuttal, those on the opposing side who argue on behalf of the rights of patients to choose any treatments, even irrational treatments, will express a number of concerns, in particular that granting physicians the power to withhold treatment on the grounds of medical futility will reverse recent gains in patient's rights against medical paternalism. They also will caution that physicians could use futility as an excuse to arbitrarily abandon patients in covert acts of rationing or for other unethical reasons. Sadly, this debate distracts the medical team from concentrating their efforts on all the possibilities of comfort care it can provide to dying patients in the final days and hours of life.

BEYOND FUTILITY TO AN ETHIC OF CARE

In this narrow debate we, together with Dr. Kathy Faber-Langendoen, have argued that a crucial element has been overlooked, both at the bedside and in public commentary. The physician has an ethical duty to redirect efforts from life-saving treatments toward the aggressive pursuit of treatments that maximize comfort and dignity for the patient and for the grieving family.[15]

An *ethic of care* has a long-standing and prominent place in the history of medicine,[16] summarized nicely in the fifteenth century French adage, "to cure sometimes, to relieve often, to comfort always." Unfortunately, the historical development of scientific medicine and the rising status of physicians has put physicians at odds with such activities as patient empathy and care. Little in their training today is devoted to improving their abilities of engagement and identification with others.

We find an ethic of care most clearly articulated in the nursing literature, where it is defined as a commitment to protecting and enhancing the patient's dignity.[17] Caring goes beyond good intentions or simple kindness and includes psychological, philosophic or religious, and physical components, taking into consideration the patient's social context and specific goals. And although "caring" is used in different ways, we use this term to refer specifically to emotional connections between persons that include affective, cognitive, and volitional dimensions. All three aspects are important. An *affective* dimension is key to caring because unless one actually "feels with" the person, pleased and relieved when the person is doing well, worried or anxious when the person is not, one does not really care. A *cognitive* component is essential, since merely feeling concerned is not sufficient; one must also have knowledge and understanding of the other person's needs, welfare, and circumstances. Finally, a *volitional* dimension is necessary to caring, since to care means not only to want what is good for another, but to act in bringing this about.[18]

The concept of palliative care, which emphasizes the relief of symptoms and the easing of pain, is becoming increasingly accepted by physicians and used in acute-care hospitals, in designated palliative care units, and in institutional and home-based hospice programs.

The call to emphasize an ethic of care when disease can no longer be cured or controlled requires strengthening collaborative efforts among health care professionals. Already, physicians and nurses have much to learn from one another, as well as from experts in hospice care and those who are conducting research into ways to improve palliative care.[19] For example, physicians owe to hospice nurses the discovery that treatments aimed at keeping dying patients well hydrated with intravenous fluids often *add* to patient discomfort by worsening respiratory secretions and dyspnea.[20] And contrary to popular perceptions of neglect if patients are allowed to die without tubes in their veins and gut, forcing carbohydrate-containing foods and fluids in well-meaning efforts to prevent "starvation" in fact *prevents* the sedative and euphoric effects of metabolic acidosis.[21]

Changing these public perceptions will require active educational efforts by health professionals. We believe that health professionals should also be advocates for creating institutional facilities that permit patients the option of dying in the privacy and presence of loved ones and friends, rather than in the far more usual (and impersonal) setting of intensive care units, surrounded by the instruments of high technology and bustling and intrusive hospital providers. Making these alternatives available—giving patients and families these choices—will be achieved, we hope, by any new national health care plan's reimbursement for home-based and hospice services.

While an ethic of care is sometimes seen as coming into force only when cure can no longer be expected, it is fitting that the French dictum was to comfort *always*. A view of medicine that sees care and cure as diametrically opposed values ill-serves patients who need compassion and relief of troubling symptoms even in the midst of potentially curative therapy. However, when medical intervention is futile in achieving the goals of curing or ameliorating disease, the comfort of the patient rises to the fore as the primary attainable goal. As it assumes this primacy, all medical interventions can be critically examined to see if they contribute to the patient's comfort, and those that do not aid the patient's comfort ought to be discarded.

Finally, better caring for patients when medical treatment is futile calls for public education and improved communication between health professionals and patients. As Dr. Timothy Quill has noted, "Sharing feelings . . . with an empathic listener can be the first step toward healing. At [the very] least, isolation is taken out of the doubt and despair."[22] Sitting down and talking with the patient helps to give voice to the patient's concerns and fears, validate the patient's feelings, educate the patient about what to expect, and humanize the dying process for both the health professional and the patient. Moreover, sensitive exploration of the patient's or family's request for a futile treatment will often yield avenues of help that were previously unanticipated and that are acceptable to all parties. Fears of abandonment, for example, can be addressed by turning the family's and medical team's attention to working intensively with a dying patient to minimize pain and suffering, address psychosocial and spiritual issues, and prepare for death. And denial of death can be addressed through a counseling process that helps the patient or family to face and find meaning in the dying process. Although "merely sitting down and getting to know" the patient is derided by some physicians as "soft" medicine, or even eliminated from the physician's role altogether and delegated to other health professionals (social workers and nurses), responsible and humane medicine cannot occur without it. It is only through exploration of the latent content of requests for futile interventions that physicians can achieve medicine's goal of healing the patient.

All too often, patients demand futile treatments because of the symbolic message such treatment conveys. As a consequence, patients and families have come to feel symbolically cared for only when the most modern invasive technologies are applied. Again, images of abandonment are heard, and words such as "starvation" and "neglect" are used to describe patients who are not connected to intravenous lines, gastrostomy tubes, or ventilators. We wish to emphasize that futile interventions are poor ways of promoting caring and compassion. Futile treatments make a mockery of caring by substituting technology for human communication and touch.

Medicine, like all human enterprises, has its own inevitable limits. While these limits may shift with advances in technology and science, it is deceptive to act as though medicine can conquer all disease, or even death itself. Nor is it sufficient merely to refrain from offering or employing futile interventions that do not work. Rather, we urge that the discussion of futility move beyond definitional debates to promote a positive ethic of care, including research and educational efforts into the care of patients when those inevitable limits are reached. Overlooked in this limited perspective is a whole set of obligations that involve not only aggressive attacks on the dying process but also the physician's duty to enhance the patient's comfort and dignity maximally during the last days of life, including aggressively working to alleviate pain and suffering.

Again, we raise the point that patients and families who "demand everything" are not entitled to demand miracles of the medical profession. And again we acknowledge that medicine—through marketing and other strategies of self-promotion—has been a shameful participant in fostering miraculous expectations among the lay public. But physicians are not and have never been obligated to treat in expectation of a miracle. We would even press the argument further: Attempting futile treatments constitutes irresponsible medical practice and should be condemned by the profession.

There are innumerable goals that persons strive for in the course of living and dying. Happiness, religious peace, reconciliation with estranged family, a sense of having fought to the death with honor — these all are goals that, although laudable and brought into sharp focus by disease, are beyond the reach of medicine. Ill health and the prospect of one's death confront the individual with many perplexing problems, only some of which can be addressed by physicians' remedies. While physicians are fundamentally obligated to comfort patients, it is arrogant to pretend that physicians are equipped to fulfill every conceivable desire.[23]

HOW SHOULD PHYSICIANS RESPOND TO FAMILIES WHO WANT EVERYTHING DONE?

The physicians caring for Helga Wanglie expended great time, care, and compassion in trying to persuade the Wanglie family to allow them to discontinue what all the health care providers concluded was inappropriate medical treatment that did not serve to benefit Mrs. Wanglie. Thus in fairness to the doctors, nothing short of a declaration of medical futility, supported by societal values, would have sufficed. In many other situations, however, we have discovered that families' demands are not so intractable if the subtext of their demands are understood and addressed. In our experience, physicians and families welcome discussions that involve not only the negative act of withholding and withdrawing life-sustaining treatment but also the positive act of enhancing the last remaining days of life. These discussions should neither be confined to obtaining a simple yes or no about a particular procedure nor be typified by the physician turning all care to the nursing staff. Rather, we believe such plans should provide strategies for maximizing comfort and dignity in the waning hours and days of life within the context of all that surrounds that patient, including family and friends.

In this regard, physicians and nurses are morally obligated to use narcotics, sedatives, and other palliative measures with the same professional skill they apply to any other treatment efforts. Continuing to draw blood, insert feeding tubes, surround the patient with monitors and other invasive technologies should be avoided unless they clearly contribute to the patient's well-being. If physicians, as a profession, are granted the responsibility and authority to make determinations of medical futility, they are all the more obligated to act according to an ethic of care. In particular, this will require better collaborative, interdisciplinary efforts among all health care professionals. At present, physicians and nurses, despite generations of collaborative efforts on behalf of patients, exist in separate professional and social worlds. We believe they have much to gain from breaking down the barriers that separate them — as well as breaking down barriers between them and experts from hospice and others who are conducting research into ways to improve palliative care.

It is our hope that in the future, patients and providers who want "everything done" will direct their efforts and emotional energies not to useless treatments that serve only to magnify suffering and threaten human dignity but to treatments that work to the maximum benefit of the patient. Saying no to futile treatment does not mean saying no to caring for the patient, but rather means transferring aggressive efforts away from life *prolongation* and toward life *enhancement* in the waning hours and days of existence. Ideally, "doing everything" means optimizing the potential for a good life, then permitting that most important coda to a good life — a "good death."

CHAPTER 5

FUTILITY AND

RATIONING

The residents of the single-room-occupancy apartment noticed that Mr. Burrows (not his real name) had failed to show up for his usual morning chat down in the lobby. A neighbor went up three flights of stairs and found him spread out in bed, shaking, confused, and gasping for breath. "What's wrong, Harry?" asked the neighbor, peering into the room. The 83-year-old retired plumber only shook his head and rubbed his belly. The neighbor called 911 and soon the elderly man was spread out on another bed, this time in the emergency department. "What's wrong, Harry?" asked the resident physician. But again the man only shook his head and kept rubbing his belly.

It did not take long before Dr. Vincent (not his real name) discovered that his new patient was in shock, and had a high fever and a bladder so swollen that it caused a bulge in his abdomen. He passed a catheter into his urethra and sprung loose a large volume of cloudy, infected urine. Dr. Vincent made a diagnosis of acute urinary retention and possible gram-negative sepsis, a widespread infection that could lead rapidly to death if not treated promptly with the right antibiotic. But which antibiotic to choose? The bacteria in these circumstances could be any one of at least a dozen organisms, each of which has its own pattern of resistance to antibiotics. The young resident physician did what he had been trained to do under the circumstances: He obtained urine and blood cultures to identify the infecting organism more precisely. But for the 24 to 48 hours it would take until the laboratory completed the identification, he prescribed a cocktail of antibiotics in hopes that by chance one of them would be effective.

Only one treatment was skipped — a monoclonal antibody infusion recently developed to neutralize the toxin of one particular species of bacteria, *Escherichia coli* J5, which was known to precipitate lethal shock. Although later studies threw doubts on the first reports, a notice had gone out from the hospital pharmacy reporting a prospective, double-blind clinical study just published in the *New*

England Journal of Medicine describing a 39 percent reduction in mortality with the use of the monoclonal antibody.[1] The notice also pointed out its high cost: $4,000 per course of treatment.[2]

When Dr. Vincent presented Mr. Burrows to the doctors on rounds the next morning, one of us asked why the monoclonal antibody treatment had not been ordered. At first, Dr. Vincent said that he considered the treatment futile. Why? Well, the man's advanced age, the severity of his illness (probable gram-negative sepsis), and particularly his underlying condition (an enlarged prostate obstructing his bladder that was probably too risky for surgery to attempt to alleviate)—all these factors made his long-term outlook poor. But we reminded Dr. Vincent of the *New England Journal of Medicine* article reporting the advantages of using the monoclonal antibody to treat the acute life-threatening illness. True, Mr. Burrows might have more attacks of urinary obstruction and gram-negative sepsis in the long term, but if he recovered from this episode, he could well live for months or even years subject only to bothersome symptoms that could be treated medically. In other words, the monoclonal antibody couldn't really be regarded as *futile,* could it? No, Dr. Vincent agreed contritely, not really.

Obviously he was uncomfortable. Under gentle prodding he finally blurted out. "Look, the guy is already in his 80s. I just don't think it's right to be spending tens or what could be even hundreds of thousands of dollars on him when the best we can do is give him maybe a year or two more of poor quality of life, if that much. Meanwhile look at all the other people—kids, particularly—who have their whole life ahead of them—they're the ones we should be giving this treatment to."

The other doctors chimed in their agreement and we nodded sympathetically. "That could very well be. But how are you going to make sure the money you saved on Mr. Burrows will get spent on those people you consider more deserving?"

Dr. Vincent admitted he had no way of doing this. From this point on the discussion involving Dr. Vincent and the other doctors clarified the distinction between futility (implying no therapeutic benefits) and rationing (implying possible therapeutic benefits, but also implying concerns about cost and allocation of limited resources).

We admitted to sharing the frustration of all the others. Of course, none of us would object to providing a potentially beneficial, albeit costly, treatment to Mr. Burrows if we didn't feel that his treatment consumed limited resources and prevented others from getting the treatments they needed. And yet, we had to point out that in our "open" system of health care there was no way to shift resources from this patient to another deemed more deserving. How could we control decisions made by other doctors on other patients, who might have even *less* chance of benefit? The fact is, without a general institutional or societal policy that provided guidelines for allocating limited resources openly and fairly, the only choice we have at our disposal today is to either provide or deny Mr. Burrows the treatment he needs.

In conclusion, we encouraged Dr. Vincent to do what all concerned physicians should do: draw public attention to the serious problem of defining conditions of medical futility and rationing and urge society to take action. But right now he owed a duty to treat Mr. Burrows with whatever beneficial treatments were available.

THE DIFFERENT CONNOTATIONS OF RATIONING AND FUTILITY

It is probably more than coincidental that Dr. Vincent represented a rationed treatment as futile, rather than representing a futile treatment as an instance of rationing. Although doctors may not like to admit that nothing can be done, it was clear that Dr. Vincent felt even more uncomfortable with the notion that medical care might be withheld because it is costly or someone else deserves it more. Why did he cover his real reason for denying the patient treatment under the guise of futility?

One possible explanation lies in the historical contexts and connotations we commonly associate with rationing. Acknowledging the need to ration violates the cherished ideal that no member of society should be considered less worthy and less desirable than any other. Because rationing involves weighing the claims of different persons, it is by its very nature discriminatory. Futility, by contrast, is concerned with the benefits treatment can produce for only a single patient. It does not make comparisons between patients. And yet, a paradox is worth noting here. When physicians are confronted with a patient's succumbing to an illness despite their best efforts, when in fact the *treatment* is failing, the physicians often report to their colleagues: The *patient* failed the treatment.

Furthermore, underlying Dr. Vincent's discomfort may have been the notion that there is something sinister in the concept of rationing. Some people simplistically impute spiraling medical costs to singular malign influences—too many lawyers, too greedy doctors, too powerful insurance companies. They assume and claim that rationing could be eradicated if only the people they single out were more pure of heart. If only society, they argue, were capable of abolishing the forces of self-interest, rationing could be done away with altogether. Futility arouses quite different concerns. It suggests that there simply is nothing anyone can do—as though the doctor is merely reporting an objective fact rather than making a value-laden decision. It does not imply a failure of generosity, only a limit to human capacity.

In light of the above reflections, it is understandable why futility not infrequently functions as a subterfuge for rationing. In the case of Mr. Burrows, Dr. Vincent may have been honestly confused about rationing. Or he might have felt uncomfortable addressing his true feelings. Perhaps the idea simply was too repellent to admit—his patient might be less deserving than others of an extraordinarily expensive treatment.

THE REASONS FOR GREATER ATTENTION TO FUTILITY AND RATIONING

Why are we talking about rationing and futility at all? Why have these twin topics gained such prominence in recent years? A number of factors are no doubt responsible.

THE RISE IN HEALTH CARE COSTS

To begin with, increasing health care costs represent a growing source of public and professional concern. The price of health care has risen at a faster rate than other consumer prices. Rising costs in turn have helped to fuel increased health care expenditures. In 1992, the U.S. Commerce Department reported that health care spending accounted for more than 14 percent of the U.S. total economic output (gross domestic product), amounting to $838.5 billion.[3] This means that in 1992, one of every seven dollars in the U.S. economy was devoted to health care. The Commerce Department forecasts that unless major changes occur in the health care system, spending on health care will continue to rise 12 to 15 percent per year during the next five years. And economists connected with President Clinton's proposed "Health Security Plan" hoped that health care expenditures could be *limited* to 17 percent of the gross domestic product, which would continue to make this allocation percentage far higher than that of any other country in the world.

Comparing current figures with those of prior years helps to convey their significance. In 1960, for example, national health care expenditures represented just 5.3 percent of the gross national product, and in 1970, 7.4 percent. But by 1985, that figure had jumped to 10.7 percent. These increased health care expenditures cannot be explained by economic growth and gains in productivity alone, but have required the transfer of resources from other areas of the economy.[4]

These economic facts have led many to call for measures to "cap" health care spending. One direct response to this call for limits has been increased attention to rationing health care. Undoubtedly the debate over medical futility represents an *indirect* response to the same economic circumstances. But acknowledgment of this fact should not invalidate the search for a definition of medical futility. After all, the most attractive method of containing health care costs would be to trim the fat out of the system. Since futile therapies are, by definition, of no benefit, they should be the first to go.

On the other hand, under conditions of scarcity, even *beneficial* medical treatments may be denied. When even beneficial resources are scarce, the question is not whether to ration, but how to ration. Will it be done in an explicit fashion? Or will rationing instead proceed in a covert and unsystematic manner? In organ transplantation, for example, potential recipients greatly outnumber donors and rationing is clearly needed. Which is not to say some form of irrational rationing does not already take place—producing demonstrable variations that have nothing to do with medical appropriateness, but rather with race, class, and economics.

Even where no significant shortage exists in medical resources, or in the elementary ingredients from which medical resources are produced, money to pay for medical care is itself limited. For example, whether at 12 percent, 15 percent or 25 percent, an upper limit on the percentage of gross domestic product allocated to health care inevitably will be reached. This is because continued increases in health care spending divert public funds from other social goods, such as education, transportation, law enforcement, and the environment. Thus, medical therapies are evaluated, compared, and rationed on the basis of cost as well as benefit.

THE DEVELOPMENT OF HIGH-TECHNOLOGY MEDICINE

A second reason why the topics of futility and rationing command greater attention of late has to do with medical success and the development of high-technology medicine. By "high technology," we mean apparatus and procedures based on modern sciences, as opposed to simpler healing arts; new, as opposed to long-accepted methods; scientifically complex, as distinct from common-sense approaches; costly, rather than inexpensive treatments; and limited, rather than widespread, expertise in using a particular technique.[5]

The historically recent availability of new, effective medical technologies brings to the fore issues of both futility and rationing. Early in the development of a new technology, there will be the question of establishing whether it is effective. After a new procedure has established its effectiveness, it will often present issues of justice in the distribution of limited resources. This is due, in part, to the developer's search for ways to maximize profit and recover the high cost associated with the technology's research, development, and delivery. The developer's marketing strategy will often involve promoting new applications for the technology. Each new technology inevitably competes with others for hospital space, insurance coverage, and trained personnel. In the beginning, the number of health professionals trained to apply a new technique in the clinical setting may be limited. As more health care providers are trained, they inevitably seek out more patients on whom to apply their new medical advance. Thus, when a new technology appears on the scene, it almost always is rationed, at first because it is limited, later as it becomes more widespread, because its expanded application is found to be costly and only marginally beneficial for certain groups of patients. Such rationing rarely takes place explicitly and according to publicly stated criteria, but more often implicitly and without acknowledgment and deliberation.

After a new technology becomes more widely available, therefore, the ethical problems it raises may turn from that of justly distributing a scarce medical resource to that of limiting its inappropriate use. Enthrallment with new techniques, together with the prestige sometimes associated with them and entrepreneurial pressures, may encourage excessive use, thereby exacerbating the ethical problem of using technologies under futile circumstances. In medicine this is a recurrent story: Initially a new technique is employed on a limited group of patients who can be shown clearly to benefit. Soon, however, the "indications" for the technique expand. More patients "qualify" whose benefits are only marginal. (This is sardonically referred to as the "hammer and nail" phenomenon: to the hammer, every problem is a nail.) For example, renal dialysis—which was a dramatic technology originally developed to provide life-support for patients until they recovered from temporary kidney failure—now is far more often used to keep alive patients whose kidney failure is permanent. This expansion of the technology was explicitly (albeit perhaps impulsively) sanctioned by society when Congress enacted the End Stage Kidney Disease funding program. What society did *not* sanction or even envision, however, are the many uses of renal dialysis that take place today, including keeping alive unconcious patients in a permanent vegetative state, who will never perceive any benefit, and advanced metastatic cancer patients who will never be well enough to leave the intensive care unit.

Another good example of technology with expanding indications is cardiopulmonary resuscitation (CPR). Again, this procedure originally was developed for patients with acute transient and largely reversible medical conditions, such as sudden cardiac or respiratory arrest. Today, though, CPR is applied to any number of patients who experience a cardiac arrest, regardless of their underlying disease or quality of life.[6] Indeed, in many states it *must* be employed unless patients explicitly refuse it. In New York State until 1992 this resulted in the absurd situation that all patients who were incapable of refusing CPR, *including patients in permanent vegetative state,* had to be attacked with resuscitation efforts unless they happened to have a surrogate decision-maker or to have left specific legal instructions to the contrary—which only a small fraction of patients ever had the foresight to execute.

This policy of "presumed demand" for CPR prompted medical ethicists Tom Tomlinson (a philosopher) and Howard Brody (a physician) to ask why CPR had to be attempted indiscriminately rather than viewed like any other treatment.[7] In their view, the decision to withhold CPR on grounds of medical futility is a judgment that falls within the physician's professional and technical expertise. As with any other treatment, they argue, it should be offered only if it can benefit the patient.

In contrast to rationing, the main thrust of this appeal is not that resources or staff are limited, but that treatment is not medically beneficial. Naturally, skeptics may wonder, "Is futility invoked to disguise rationing? Would the issue of futility be raised in the absence of competition for limiting resources?"

THE AGING OF SOCIETY

A third element encouraging greater focus on futility and rationing is the aging of society. Although the population of most developed countries has been aging since 1800, the pace of aging has accelerated greatly in recent years. Since 1900, for example, the United States has witnessed an eightfold increase in the number of people over the age of 65. Those over the age of 85, the fastest-growing age group in the country, are 21 times as numerous as in 1900. The elderly are also the heaviest users of health services. Persons 65 and over represent approximately 12 percent of the U.S. population, but account for about one third of the nation's total personal health care expenditures, exclusive of research costs.

The phenomenon of an aging society has led some to question public funding of life-extending health care in old age. "Today, about 2% of Gross Domestic Product goes to Medicare payments for people who are within six months of dying," says Allan Meltzer, an economist at Carnegie Mellon University, who adds bluntly, "And I think that is a waste."[8] According to ethicist Daniel Callahan, even if life-extending medical care were unlimited, elderly people themselves would be wise to settle for the achievement of a limited natural lifespan.[9] The suggestion is not that public investments in life-extending therapies for older individuals produce no medical benefit; rather, these treatments are futile in a broad sense: death in old age is inevitable and an acceptance of limits is therefore fitting. (This, in fact, is the argument Dr. Vincent was initially pressing.)

This broad sense of futility should not be confused with our own definition. Callahan's definition is not based on medical criteria, such as the poor likelihood of achieving medical benefits for older patients or the low quality of medical benefits in older age groups. Indeed, such an approach would be difficult to sustain, as evidence is mounting that no significant age difference exists in mortality or morbidity outcomes associated with various interventions, including survival after CPR for in-hospital cardiac arrests and coronary arteriography, liver and kidney transplantation and other surgeries, chemotherapy and dialysis.[10] Rather than basing his concept of futility on medical criteria, Callahan's approach is strictly age-based, drawing a line at an upper age limit. By contrast, we define futility in terms of medical outcomes and perceive no necessary correlation between the futility of an intervention and the age of a patient.

Despite the lack of evidence showing that older individuals consistently experience poorer medical outcomes, elderly people recently have become a target for denial of care based on rationing as well as futility. The appeal of age-based rationing is due in part to the fact that the ranks of older Americans are swelling, and the cost of care for elderly people is disproportionately high. While not all agree that rationing health care based on age is ethically or philosophically sound, several arguments have been advanced in support of such a proposal. Productivity arguments hold that the goal of maximizing life-years saved, or costs saved, or contributions to the public good, can best be achieved by limiting the health care to elderly people. Other arguments claim that if individuals, such as our patient, Mr. Burrows, were to view their lives as a whole, rather than at a particular moment in time, their considered preferences would be to distribute more medical resources to earlier, rather than later, years.[11]

LIMITS ON PATIENT AUTONOMY

A final basis for greater attention to futility and rationing has been a growing tendency to restrict patient autonomy. Since the early

1960s, the principle of patient autonomy has dominated the field of bioethics, and physician paternalism has been replaced by an ethic of respect for the choices of competent patients. Autonomy has been trumpeted by ethicists like Robert Veatch as an overriding ethical value, essentially canceling out other moral values, such as beneficence, when they conflict with it.[12]

However, the principle of radical autonomy has recently been challenged from a variety of sources. Although some continue to insist that patients are entitled to care that is medically useless or only marginally medically beneficial, other ethicists are beginning to hold physicians ethically responsible for *refraining* from offering or continuing futile treatment. Allan Brett and Laurence McCullough, for example, argue that when a patient seeks to exercise a right to medical care, a necessary condition is that there is either an established or theoretical *medical* basis for the patient's request.[13] In the absence of at least a modicum of medical benefit, they argue, the whole point of the physician–patient interaction disappears. Others maintain that the moral authority to make decisions regarding futile resuscitation does not rest exclusively with the patient or family but rather with the community of medicine, which is entitled to establish a professional consensus about the purposes to which their skills will be put. For example, based on a growing literature on the outcomes of medical treatments applied to specific patient groups, physicians and ethicists have argued that physicians should withhold or refrain from offering certain treatments in a range of cases: CPR to patients with overwhelming burn injury; patients without a reasonable chance of discharge from an intensive care unit; patients with no chance of recovery from CPR; patients whose lives will not be preserved or suffering alleviated; severely ill infants incapable of experiencing pain and whose prognosis is poor and survival questionable; terminally ill incompetent patients, even those whose families request aggressive treatments.[14]

Another source of challenge to allowing patient autonomy to trump all opposing arguments is that health care resources are scarce and may be exhausted long before patients' demands for those resources can be met. Many have begun to argue that the health care provider's ethical role now requires balancing justice in the distribution of resources against the responsibility to advocate for individual patients' interests. While some continue to press for health care professionals to devote their energies exclusively to meeting patients' requests and promoting patients' welfare, many now hold that physicians do not owe patients a level of resources beyond what patients are entitled to receive, nor must physicians sacrifice their honor, professional integrity, or personal welfare in order to satisfy patients' demands. Others argue that patients' requests should be checked, either by placing physician-patient relationships in the context of institutions that guarantee a fair distribution of resources or by instituting socially sound public policies. Reflecting these sentiments, the President's Commission, in its 1983 report, *Securing Access to Health Care,* acknowledged that the health care system, like every other system for organizing an activity,

> places some limitations on individual choice. . . . Thus, the issue is what kinds of limitations on choice are most consistent with fulfilling society's moral obligation to provide equitable access to health care for all . . . since an adequate level is something less than all care that might be beneficial, patients' choices will be limited to that range unless they are able to pay for care that exceeds adequacy.[15]

The common historical, demographic, economic, and ethical background of futility and rationing makes evident that it will not be possible to keep futility judgment and rationing judgment completely distinct. Whenever the futility of a treatment is debated, its economic cost is also likely to be lurking in the background of the discussion. This hardly shows, however, that the two concepts mean the same thing, or provide the same ethical warrant for withholding or withdrawal of medical treatment. As we shall argue in the next sections, futility and rationing have both common and distinguishing features. Although standards for rationing of very low-benefit treatment are likely to be an important part of health care reform, we have argued that futile treatments should not be offered even if they were (hypothetically) cheap and abundant.

COMMON FEATURES OF FUTILITY AND RATIONING

To return to our patient, Mr. Burrows, it is important to say that the tendency for the physician to confuse futility and rationing is not unusual. On the contrary, since attention to futility and rationing has occurred simultaneously, the two concepts are frequently confused by health care providers and others. Thus, it may be helpful to set forth both the common and distinguishing features.

Futility and rationing share a common ground in situations in which rationing is based on either the quality or likelihood of medical benefit. First, in situations in which rationing assigns a low priority to persons who have the poorest quality of medical outcome, treatment may also be withheld based on a judgment that the *quality* of a particular medical outcome is so extraordinarily poor that it is futile. To state that the quality of outcome is medically futile is to judge that the result achieved by a therapeutic intervention falls below a minimal medical outcome threshold. That is, if the best result the treatment can achieve is so poor, the treatment should be regarded as futile and not attempted.

Similarly, rationing that rests on the low likelihood that a medical benefit will occur bears a resemblance to futility assessment based on the poor chance of achieving a certain outcome. Again, medical futility in this sense expresses the idea that the likelihood of achieving an acceptable medical goal is below a threshold considered minimal.

A final resemblance between futility and rationing concerns the manner in which such decisions are reached and implemented. This can range from clearly stated to never articulated, publicly defended to covertly accomplished, and ethically supported to ethically indefensible.

A particularly striking example of the common features of futility and rationing occurred in President Clinton's proposed "Health Security Plan."[16] Under the president's plan, health care treatments not deemed "necessary and appropriate" were excluded from the basic package of health care benefits that all health care plans were required to provide. The president proposed appointing a national health board to decide which treatments fall under the heading of "unnecessary and inappropriate." Thus, the president's plan would ration health care treatments under circumstances where they are judged to provide only a marginal quality or likelihood of benefit — and thus are not costworthy. However, in some instances, the quality or likelihood of benefit associated with the excluded treatment-condition pairs may be so small that the particular application of the treatment could also be regarded as medically futile. Commenting on the role of the National Health Board in Clinton's proposal, Ronald Dworkin noted: "Many politicians and some doctors say that much of the new technology is 'unnecessary' or 'wasteful.' They do not mean that it provides no benefit at all. . . . Heroic transplants that rarely work do work rarely. So we cannot defend the decision the . . . board would make as simply avoiding waste. We cannot avoid the question . . . what is 'appropriate' medical care. . . ."[17] Although we agree with Dworkin that despite low odds of success, some quantitatively futile treatments may benefit (but remember— also harm) the patient, we do not agree that the question of their medical appropriateness is therefore left open and insoluble. In contrast, we have argued that health professionals have a professional obligation *not* to provide inappropriate interventions. In our view, if a particular application of a treatment has been shown to have such an exceedingly low chance of success that common sense (and a medical and societal consensus) deem it futile, then it would be medically inappropriate to offer the treatment.

Indeed, we are concerned that for some who enter the debate on medical futility, "it's only a matter of money," implying that medicine should take its place next to the "oldest profession" and "do anything" as long as someone is willing to pay for it. The pervasiveness of this perspective was evident in the media coverage of the Baby K case, an anencephalic infant (born with most of her brain congenitally absent) who had been kept alive by medical technology for more than a year (see Chapter 10). The hospital wanted to stop further medical treatment, but the mother went to court demanding that maximal emergency medical care and life support be continued. "Court Order To Treat Baby Prompts a Debate on Ethics" the *New York Times* declared on February 20, 1994. But the sub-headline ("At What Point Does Treatment Cease to Be Worth the Expense?") indicated that as far as the newspaper was concerned, the debate was not about whether physicians should be keeping alive a body with no possibility of human existence, but rather whether that enterprise was worth the money. Is that the moral code and professional standard society wishes to assign to medicine? Is that the way physicians see themselves—willing to do anything as long as someone offers to pay for it?

To illustrate the common features of futility and rationing, consider the following case on which one of us was asked to serve as an ethics consultant.

Juanita was an 8-year-old Mexican girl with acute lymphocytic leukemia. Her mother would transport her across the border to a university medical center in the United States whenever her daughter began to lose weight and become severely weak. The university hospital doctors who made the original diagnosis and prescribed the chemotherapy treated her even though they knew she was not a U.S. citizen and could not afford to pay. Each time they advised her mother to continue follow-up treatment in Mexico. Instead, every few months they saw the girl, each time with her disease in an advanced stage of relapse. The woman claimed she was unable to obtain the necessary treatment in her own country.

This time the hematologists faced a situation that was particularly grim. The disease was now resistant to the available chemotherapy drugs, and any more radical treatment such as bone marrow transplantation was hazardous and expensive and no longer promising. The mother—who had relentlessly pursued what she regarded as the best treatment in the United States—pleaded with the doctors to do everything possible to save her daughter's life. The doctors were in a quandary. Since they knew the mother and daughter from previous encounters, they had begun to feel a special relationship with them. And of course, they wanted to save Juanita's life if they could.

What should they do? It was clear at this point that even the most aggressive treatments had an exceedingly small chance of saving her life. But were the chances so vanishingly small as to consider all treatment futile? While sorting that out among themselves, they could not ignore a further consideration. She was not a citizen of the United States. In other words, if one were to ask whether or not she was entitled to the treatment, one would clearly have to consider the matter of distributive justice.

In a just society one seeks to achieve a fair distribution of benefits and burdens. In the case of Juanita, the benefits were obviously medical treatments that could save her life. But neither she nor anyone in her family had participated in sharing the burdens, namely taxes that go to pay for hospital care. (Ironically, of course, if they were as poor in the United States as they were in Mexico, they probably would not have had sufficient income to pay taxes in comparison to the welfare support they received. But still, they would have been exposed to the obligations of tax burdens.)

In this example, the question of whether to provide Juanita a bone marrow transplant raises issues of both rationing and futility. With respect to *rationing,* one concern is the low likelihood or quality of benefit, and the consideration that other patients stand to benefit more from a similar investment of resources. The basis for futility also involves evaluating the potential benefits of treatment. If the likelihood or quality of benefit Juanita would receive from the transplant fails to approach a threshold considered minimal, then the transplant can be withheld on grounds of futility as well as rationing.

DISTINGUISHING FEATURES OF FUTILITY AND RATIONING

Despite the commonality of meaning between futility and rationing, several distinctions can be noted. Foremost is that futility has no explicit distributive meaning, that is, it does not involve making comparisons across a large number of patients, but instead refers to a specific cause-and-effect logic in a single patient. Thus, although rationing based on quality or probability of medical benefit partially overlaps with futility, a difference remains. Whereas rationing indicates a priority *among* scarce resources, futility implies that a *particular* medical intervention produces an unacceptably low likelihood or quality of benefit. Thus, in the case of Mr. Burrows or Juanita, the judgment of medical futility had to come down to: Is there at least a reasonable chance that the treatment would achieve an acceptable medical outcome *in this patient,* regardless of who else might deserve it more or derive greater benefit?

A second point of contrast between futility and rationing is that criteria for rationing are far broader in scope than are criteria for defining futility. For example, it might be argued that we should ration based on standards such as age, citizenship, ability to pay, social utility, or equality. However, no one could intelligibly argue that medical treatment is futile on these grounds. The patient could be old or young, a citizen of the United States or Mexico. None of these factors per se affects the potential benefit of the treatment. Strictly speaking, medically futile treatment can be denied only when the patient's particular *medical* circumstances indicate that an expected outcome will fail to meet acceptable goals of medical practice.

A third, and related, point is that ethical rationing must meet standards articulated in theories of distributive justice, namely, theories that indicate what is a fair distribution of burdens and benefits within a society. By contrast, the manner of determining and justifying criteria of medical futility does not make reference to justice theories. Instead, the medical and lay communities have to look to general professional opinion about such things as medical indications and community values and goals. In other words, if a standard of care regarding medical futility is to be established it must be decided by a broad consensus among health professionals and others. A good model to follow here is the evolution to the present definition of death in terms of brain-death criteria. In the 1960s, with the advent of cardiac pacemakers and ventilators, the definition of death became ambiguous and disputed; however, critical ethical debate resulted in a convergence of opinion and consistent policy. We urge that equally vigorous efforts be made to define medical futility. If we fail to exert such efforts and to achieve agreement about the definition of medical futility, this will only invite a confusing and, in our opinion, seriously harmful patchwork of case law decisions and inconsistent policies. "Roving strangers" will be tempted to run from hospital to hospital and state to state looking for Mr. Burrowses and Juanitas to push their singular moral agendas into the resulting ethical and legal vacuums.

A final difference between futility and rationing is that the circumstances of rationing always presuppose scarcity. By contrast, it is possible to argue for denying futile treatment even where a resource is abundant and cheap. For example, even though cough medicine is cheap and abundant, the doctors taking care of Mr. Burrows and Juanita wouldn't even consider prescribing it, for the simple reason that it would not alleviate the medical problems.

THE PSYCHOLOGICAL ROOTS OF FUTILITY AND RATIONING

One fact is undeniable: We are reluctant to embrace either rationing or futility with open arms. Both are rude awakenings to medicine.

Futility forces medicine to come down from its pedestal. Its lesson to medicine is, "Doctor, you are powerless in the face of this calamity." Like Sisyphus whose repeated efforts were leading nowhere, modern doctors too often continue frantically with medical treatments well past their point of usefulness. Yet such efforts ultimately make no progress in benefiting the patient or curing the disease.

Rationing carries a different message for medicine, but one that also teaches about human limits. It announces loudly, "Doctor there is something you can do but we won't let you." Rationing puts someone else in charge. It ties doctors' hands by putting the resources they ask for beyond their reach. Like Odysseus, who heard the sirens but was tied to the mast and prevented from reaching them, the modern doctor is tethered to resource constraints and oversight committees. Yet the analogy between the doctor and Odysseus is not exact, for Odysseus requested to be tied and swore to himself that he would not give in to the sirens' alluring song. Odysseus's restraint therefore showed his self-restraint. Modern physicians, by contrast, are obviously chafing under the restraints imposed on them. Their training teaches them to do everything possible to promote patients' interests. Cost-containment is not yet one of the subjects taught in medical school; its lessons come from the outside, causing doctors to feel hemmed in. They feel inclined, even obligated, to somehow break free. Physicians do not yet define their role as incorporating social responsibilities, or perhaps they do not perceive present resource constraints as just standards for allocating health care.[18]

Just as futility and rationing shake loose the very foundations of medicine by challenging the physician's control and mastery, so too they shake *society* by challenging its relentless faith in science and medicine. Rationing gives the unmistakable message that not everyone enjoys the fruit of medicine's labor. (Recall how often during debates on health care reform, politicians irresponsibly incant the word *rationing* in order to strike fear in the mind of the public—as though rationing does not already exist.) Futility reminds society that, despite the great strides science has made, its knowledge and power are ultimately limited.

These messages are all the more ominous when life-saving medical treatment is at stake. Rationing life-saving treatments implies that even life itself is not of unconditional value; even life is not something we will purchase at any price. Here, rationing's message is not simply that we cannot have it all, but that we must make the ultimate sacrifice. The withdrawal of a futile life-sustaining treatments conveys an equally unattractive thought: when life itself is on the line, all of the sophisticated methods of science may be powerless to save it.

As we have already pointed out, the harsh message futility carries can be softened only when medicine places greater emphasis and value on caring for patients. Saying no to futile treatments is consistent with continuing to nurture and provide comfort to patients. Unfortunately, however, "in American medicine ideals of heroic achievement increasingly have overshadowed the value of nurturance. . . . Technological advances repeatedly have been gained at the expense of the doctor-patient relationship."[19] We believe that this state of affairs is not inevitable, that recognizing futility challenges physicians to alter it.

With respect to rationing, a similar point is in order. Saying no to costly medical therapies should be compatible with showing respect for persons. Yet this will occur only when rationing is tempered by justice. Rationing can be palatable only provided that it takes place under conditions in which everyone enjoys access to basic services.[20]

We submit that the challenge for medicine, indeed for all of us, is to not to recoil by evading hard choices, but instead to realize the limits of medicine in a manner that still preserves, even strengthens, our sense of compassion and community.

CHAPTER 6

MEDICAL

FUTILITY IN

A LITIGIOUS

SOCIETY

One summer day in 1988, 6-month-old Sammy Linares attended his last birthday party. In the midst of the festivities, he choked on a deflated balloon. By the time his father, Rudy Linares, noticed what had happened, the baby was already blue and unconscious. Frantically the father attempted mouth-to-mouth resuscitation, then picked the child up and ran half a block to a neighborhood fire station for help. There firefighters managed to remove the balloon and continued efforts at resuscitation. But not until the boy was taken by ambulance to the McNeil Hospital Emergency Room were doctors and nurses able to reestablish the baby's pulse and blood pressure. By then an estimated twenty minutes had elapsed between the baby's asphyxia and the return of his own spontaneous heartbeat.

For the remaining nine months of his life in the Rush Presbyterian St. Lukes Medical Center Pediatric Intensive Care Unit, the heart continued to beat, but Sammy Linares never regained consciousness. Again and again the physicians attempted to withdraw the ventilator, but the baby's brain damage was too severe to allow him to breathe on his own. Reluctantly, the physicians concluded that the baby would never recover consciousness and never survive off the ventilator. At this point, Rudy Linares asked that the ventilator be disconnected so that his baby son could die.

All of the doctors and nurses caring for the baby agreed with the father that there was no point in continuing to keep the permanently unconscious body alive. But even though there were precedents both in ethics and the law to allow life support to be withdrawn under these circumstances,[1] the physicians chose to seek the opinion of the hospital's legal counsel. His response is worth recording: "What we are dealing with here is a legal problem."[2]

Not a medical problem, a legal problem. This astonishing statement reveals how impoverished the notion of medical professional responsibility has become. Before agreeing to discontinue the ventilator, the hospital demanded that the Linares family obtain a court order. Why were the hospital authorities unwilling to go to court themselves if they truly believed in the appropriateness of the request and were simply seeking legal protection? The only explanation is that the best interests of the patient were overshadowed by the hospital's concern for its public image. The Linares family had already cost the state's Medicaid program over half a million dollars. Wouldn't the hospital be vulnerable to the tabloid press if it was sensationalized as a killer of welfare babies? Rather than risk its reputation, the hospital was prepared to keep the unconscious baby alive indefinitely.

Meanwhile, Rudy Linares kept repeating his request that the baby be allowed to die in peace. Once, while visiting his son in the middle of the night, he disconnected the ventilator himself, but security guards wrestled him to the ground and the medical staff reconnected the machine.

After nine months the distraught father took a more desperate step in carrying out his wishes. Following one of their visits, he sent his wife away and suddenly produced a gun. Holding the intensive care unit staff at bay and saying "I'm not here to hurt anyone," he disconnected his son's respirator and waited for the boy to die. As proof that he meant no harm, he allowed the hospital staff to remove three other patients from the intensive care unit. Then, after confirming the baby's death with a stethoscope that a physician slid across the floor, Rudy Linares surrendered to police.

To the hospital staff's astonishment, when the story reached the press they had so feared, the public outrage was directed against them—not against Mr. Linares. The state's attorney filed a murder complaint, requiring Rudy Linares to undergo a psychiatric evaluation as a condition of his bond, but a grand jury refused to issue a homicide indictment. In the end Rudy Linares was found guilty only of a misdemeanor weapons charge. Indeed, many of us in the field of medical ethics thought that the only crime for which Mr. Linares could be found guilty was practicing medicine without a license. For Mr. Linares, in his own clumsy, desperate way, was trying to do what all the doctors and nurses wanted to do—*thought they ought to do*—but failed to do.

FEAR OF LAWYERS

In this chapter we will explore the interactions of medicine and the law, particularly with respect to establishing standards of care determining medical futility. But first we must acknowledge the immense presence of the law in contemporary American society. A few statistics can serve. Between 1960 and 1990 the number of lawyers in this country nearly tripled, from 260,000 to 756,000. Although the ratio of lawyers to the general population remained fairly constant at about 120 per 100,000 Americans until 1970, now that ratio is more than 300 lawyers per 100,000—the highest in the world. In the area of health care, lawyers have not only played a role in provoking what is commonly referred to as "defensive medicine," but have influenced every aspect of health care delivery. For example, the number of health care lobbying groups, heavily populated with lawyers and affecting legislation at every level of government, has soared from 117 in 1979 to 741 in 1991.[3]

Whether the medical malpractice system adversely influences the behavior of physicians, causing them to prescribe tests and treatments whose principal aim is to protect physicians from lawsuits rather than protect their patients from disease, it is a subject of continuing controversy. Unfortunately the latest evidence suggests that fear of liability does distort the practice of medicine. How serious is the distortion? Certainly it is costly. Recently the American Medical Association estimated that physicians spent $15.1 billion in 1989 for marginal or unnecessary tests and procedures solely (and often misguidedly) to protect themselves from malpractice suits. This is in addition to $5.6 billion spent on professional liability insurance premiums. And although costs incurred and harms caused by overutilization cannot be separated easily from other influences (such as financial incentives and restrictions, patient preferences for aggressive treatments, peer review organization requirements and prevailing notions of safety and efficacy), analysts have concluded that "defensive medicine is a real phenomenon accounting for at least some marginal or unnecessary care."[4]

For example, it has been more than twenty years since researchers investigated whether obtaining skull X-rays on all patients admitted to the emergency room with head injuries would lead to the discovery of clinically undetectable skull fractures. After reviewing the results of 1,500 X-rays, the researchers concluded that for a certain group of 435 patients, obtaining skull X-rays added very little to information that wasn't already obtained by simply questioning and examining the patients. Only one of the patients in this easily defined group had an undetected fracture. The researchers suggested that skull X-rays of patients whose clinical findings fit into the low-yield group could be omitted without causing any undue damage.[5]

From a medical perspective, therefore, continuing to perform a skull X-ray on *all* emergency room patients with head injury would seem unreasonable, particularly in certain clinically defined circumstances. And from a societal perspective millions of dollars could be saved if the recommendation were adopted nationwide. But what about the legal perspective? Might that one exceptional case out of any future 435 patients be viewed by a jury—under the prodding of a personal injury lawyer—to have suffered the effects of "medical negligence"? Depending on the jury's sympathy, the patient might collect hundreds of thousands, perhaps even millions, of dollars in damages, thereby wiping out all the savings produced by eliminating the X-ray, in other words by rational, sensible medical care. In any event, the study had no perceptible influence on the nation's emergency physicians, who continue to order skull X-rays unencumbered by any rational policy.

More recently, in 1988, the American College of Obstetricians and Gynecologists dropped its long-standing policy requiring electronic fetal monitoring of all pregnant women and declared that it was no longer necessary for the majority of low-risk women. But once again, the majority of obstetricians continue to use this expensive technology "despite overwhelming evidence that it does not improve neonatal mortality and morbidity rates."[6] Why? According to Peter Huber, an expert on liability law, "Lawyers have discovered in EFM [electronic fetal monitoring] the perfect technological wand to wave before juries."[7]

Indeed, the courts have shown an infatuation not only with modern technology but with outright fraudulent treatments, particularly those purported to be cancer cures, like Laetrile, immunoaugmentive therapy, and thermography. One review of court cases initiated by patients seeking insurance coverage for the costs of these treatments observed that, rather than relying on peer-reviewed scientific literature, interpreted if necessary by impartial experts, the courts often relied on "testimony by practitioners who either were the attending physician of the insured or had a vested interest in coverage of the subject procedures."[8] Astonishingly, testimonies tainted by conflict of interest that would disqualify any claim of scientific objectivity *took precedence* in these legal deliberations. Is it any wonder that physicians seeking to practice careful, rational medicine despair of achieving this goal in a legal environment so appallingly misguided at times in scientific and medical matters? The recent U.S. Supreme Court decision *Daubert v. Merrell Dow,* which assigns to the trial judge "the task of ensuring that an expert's testimony both rests on a reliable foundation and is relevant to the task at hand," may alleviate this problem, but it is too early to say.[9]

More recently, a survey of hospitals in New York State revealed the curious finding that the number of caesarean sections performed in the different hospitals varied directly with the number of malpractice claims. Since there was no significant association between caesarean deliveries and malpractice claims for individual physicians *within* each hospital, the researchers concluded that the quality of practice was not leading to the malpractice claims, but rather the other way around: the physicians' *fear* of malpractice suits was causing them to increase their tendency to perform the surgical procedure.[10]

As Huber points out, "in technology-intensive professions like medicine or aviation, there will *always* be a spare high-tech instrument, heroic procedure, or exotic medicine lying around that could have been tried, that might conceivably have made things turn out better." He adds caustically:

> The cautionary CAT scan or caesarean, the amniocentesis, blood test, or fetal monitor can be certified as essential by lawyers much faster than by scientists. These tests and gadgets then accumulate in the cockpit and the operating theater, because not having them on hand has become legally risky. As the unnecessary or unreliable tests and technologies multiply, so do the opportunities for ignoring them in the heat of a crisis. Which creates opportunities for still more legal action.[11]

It is important that society recognize this dilemma: the efforts of the medical profession to practice a reasonable, common-sense, not to mention cost-effective, medicine by eliminating unnecessary tests and futile treatments on the grounds of empirical evidence leave the profession vulnerable to legal attack in the rare and exceptional case. This conflict has implications with respect to both causing harm to patients as well as imposing costs on society, and underlies the importance of the medical profession's proactive involvement in establishing clearly defined standards of care, standards that society at large finds acceptable and the courts heed. It also illustrates the importance of educating the public (and juries) that the reasonable practice of medicine is not without unavoidable and unfortunate outcomes. If the public insists that doctors perform every conceivable test or treatment in every situation, they will be exchanging the small chance that a benefit might be missed for the greater chance that much harm will result—through side effects of the tests and treatments, as well as the side effects of additional tests administered due to false-positive findings.

This is not an idle speculation. A recent attempt to study the effectiveness of high dose chemotherapy with bone marrow transplantation to treat breast cancer ran up against unexpected obstacles. Even though there is no evidence the controversial and burdensome and highly expensive treatment is more effective than conventional chemotherapy, many patients hired lawyers to force insurance companies to pay for the treatment.[12] Patients with metastatic breast cancer were unwilling to participate in clinical trials or wait for their results. They wanted the new unproven treatment *now* and fully covered by insurance. One writer described the project as illustrating the complexity of doing research "in an arena of divided physicians, desperate patients, reluctant insurers, aggressive lawyers and revenue-hungry hospitals." But in large part the blame falls on physicians who "lack the courage to say no to patients."[13]

As members of hospital ethics committees, both of us have been involved in formulating policies for withholding and withdrawing treatment. Recently, when one hospital ethics committee completed a very carefully drafted policy and submitted it to the various clinical services for their review, one physician demanded that the ethics consultant run the policy draft past some "aggressive lawyers" to see where the loopholes were. To his credit the first lawyer responded without even looking at the policy that "physicians shouldn't be practicing medicine to avoid lawsuits, they should do what is best for the patient." The ethics consultant returned with this advice to the committee and the policy was adopted without further ado.

FEARS OF THE LAW AND LEGAL MYTHS

It is ironic that doctors have forced patients and families to accept unwanted or inappropriate life-prolonging treatments out of misplaced fear of legal liability. As professor of philosophy and clinical ethics Lance Stell points out, "From *Quinlan* [in 1976] to the present, our courts have rejected the notion that physicians have a duty to preserve biological existence per se."[14] In the *Quinlan* decision, the court asserted that "the focal point of decision should be the prognosis as to the reasonable possibility of return to cognitive and sapient life, as distinguished from the forced continuance of the biological vegetative existence."[15] It is worth drawing attention to the word *reasonable,* which performs invaluable service in American jurisprudence and might serve as a guide to medical practice. In the law, even when the accused's life hangs in the balance, say, at a trial for murder, the jury is admonished to base its conviction on evidence persuasive not beyond all doubt but beyond all *reasonable* doubt. Reasonableness tempers judgment. Similarly, physicians should also temper their judgments; they are obligated to apply their skills not if there is any miraculous chance of success but where there is a reasonable possibility of success.

It is worth repeating that there has never been a single civil judgment against or criminal conviction of a physician for withdrawing life-sustaining treatment. For all the scare stories that circulate in doctors' lounges, the decision to allow a patient to die is not considered medical negligence and threatened with astronomical awards. In a paper sharply critical of the medical and legal professions whose "serious misunderstanding of the law can lead to tragic results for physicians, health care institutions, patients, and families," professor of law and ethicist Alan Meisel summarizes eight "myths about what the law permits concerning the termination of life support."[16]

Myth No. 1: "Anything that is not specifically permitted by law is prohibited." This myth, Meisel says, "is held dear not only by some health care professionals, but by the general public and by many people who ought to know better—namely lawyers." This led to the tragedy of the Linares case, as indeed the hospital counsel testified: "I told the medical staff there was a possibility they would face criminal charges." Proffering this advice, the attorney played the role of one of the "paid paranoids whose perceived function it is to conjure up worst-case hypothetical scenarios and accordingly to render the most conservative, risk-averse advice to their clients."[17]

But, as lawyer Lawrence J. Nelson and physician Ronald E. Cranford point out, "An experienced and knowledgeable attorney, particularly one dealing with physicians and hospitals should construct his or her advice on probabilities, not abstract possibilities. The practical probability in this case of a physician being prosecuted for murder was remote to the point of being nonexistent, fundamentally because the law and the facts of this situation would not support even a vaguely plausible prosecution for unlawful, malicious killing."[18]

If ignorance of the law is found among lawyers, it seems to be widespread among physicians. Indeed, ignorance of the law, along with misguided notions that equate withholding every last means of prolonging terminal life with killing, was prevalent in over 700 physicians surveyed by the Institute for Medical Humanities in Galveston.[19] Ultimately, of course, health professionals, not lawyers, treat patients. So, not unreasonably, the researchers expressed concern over the inevitable consequences of these attitudes among physicians—unnecessary suffering of patients and families and inappropriate use of scarce resources.

Myth No. 2: "Termination of life support is murder or suicide." As we have already pointed out, court decisions around the country, including the U.S. Supreme Court's *Cruzan* decision, have made it clear that termination of inappropriate or unwanted life support in a medical setting is neither murder nor suicide. The position the courts have taken is that removal of life support under these circumstances merely allows nature to take its course and that the patient's illness, not the treatment removal, causes death. Furthermore, the courts have agreed that replacing life-prolonging treatments with comfort care, namely, treatments aimed at relieving suffering, as well as any treatments that are in response to a patient's request, whether or not they result in curtailment of life, are not criminal actions.

Myth No. 3: "A patient must be terminally ill for life support to be stopped."
Although the validity of advance directives (living wills and durable
powers of attorney for health care) have in the past been limited in
many states to the period of terminal illness, today patients can issue
orders to withhold or withdraw treatments, even life-sustaining
treatments, either orally or in writing at any time. In particular, the
U.S. Supreme Court's *Cruzan* decision, although permitting a state
to apply any evidentiary standard it sees fit, granted patients the
right to refuse *any* treatment, whether or not they are suffering from
terminal illness. And in fact many courts have permitted withdrawal
of treatment in a variety of instances short of terminal illness, including severe cerebral palsy, temporary uterine bleeding, kidney failure
requiring renal dialysis, persistent vegetative state, and quadriplegia.

*Myth No. 4: "It is permissible to terminate extraordinary treatments, but not
ordinary ones."* The distinction between ordinary and extraordinary
treatments has evaporated as medical technology becomes more and
more ordinary. Once, maintaining patients through feeding tubes was
considered extraordinary; now there are those who argue that such
feeding tubes represent basic life support. Today, CPR, mechanical
ventilation, renal dialysis, and the entire panoply of intensive-care
unit treatments are undertaken as a matter of course in seriously ill
patients. Are such treatments ordinary or extraordinary? In the tradition of Catholic moral theology, extraordinary treatments were regarded as those which provided no benefit and whose burdens were
excessive. Such a distinction can apply to even the simplest measures.
Even intravenous fluids can be regarded as extraordinary if they do
nothing but maintain an unconscious or incurably suffering patient.
Today, ethicists and courts tend to measure treatments not in terms of
ordinary versus extraordinary but in terms of proportionality and
benefits versus burdens. That is, does the treatment, whatever it is,
result overall in a balance of benefits (chance of saving cognitive, sapient life or restoring function or alleviating suffering) over burdens
(pain, suffering, loss of dignity, and costs)? Are the burdens imposed
proportionate to the benefits gained? For example, is not the prolongation of life by only a few days *dis*proportionate to the imposition of
great suffering and expenditure of tens of thousands of dollars—as
occurs today in many intensive care units around the country?

Myth No. 5: "It is permissible to withhold treatment but, once started, it must be continued." Although health care providers and families recognize that emotionally, it is sometimes more difficult to discontinue a treatment that has been started, the law has clearly followed the lead of *Barber v. Los Angeles County Superior Court,*[20] which noted that any treatment may be viewed in terms of whether or not the next application of that treatment is likely to benefit the patient. The *Barber* decision deliberately drew no distinction between withholding a ventilator or discontinuing a ventilator in a patient for whom this machine provides no benefit. Obviously there is a practical as well as theoretical value to equating withholding and withdrawing futile treatments. Physicians who are fearful of having to "pull the plug" at some later time might be tempted to avoid starting a desperate life-saving procedure. Unfortunately this misguided fear might lead them to make hasty decisions with insufficient knowledge or time to reflect, and paradoxically to *withhold* potentially beneficial treatments. For example, a patient brought into the emergency room might be an uncertain candidate for cardiopulmonary resuscitation or immediate ventilation. If the physician were to start these procedures and if they turned out to be beneficial they could of course be continued. If, on the other hand, they turned out to be inappropriate, they could *then* be discontinued. But what if the physician—to avoid facing difficult decisions—never gave the patient a "fighting chance"?

Myth No. 6: "Stopping tube feeding is legally different from stopping other treatments." The usual concern of those who seek to distinguish tube feeding from other forms of medical treatment is that patients should not be allowed to "starve to death." Yet as clinical experience has evolved (and as we have discussed in previous chapters), health professionals have learned that providing nutrition and hydration to patients who are terminally ill often adds to their suffering rather than reduces it. Moreover artificially prolonging life by any measures beyond the patient's own choice runs the risk of violating that patient's autonomy. Thus, throughout this country and finally in the U.S. Supreme Court *Cruzan* decision, most courts have held that there is no legal distinction between the termination of artificial nutrition and hydration and other forms of treatment.

Myth Number 7: "Termination of life support requires going to court." The persistence of this common misperception attests to the pervasive power of the "litigious society." It is a notion all the more absurd—if the word were not too inexpressive of the suffering caused—when one contemplates the multitude of decisions made every day by physicians that in effect terminate life-sustaining treatments. Every time a surgeon decides against performing a desperate operation, the surgeon has chosen the certainty that the patient will die over the possibility of rescuing the patient. Every time a physician prescribes high doses of a narcotic to alleviate pain in a dying patient, the physician has chosen a course of action that might shorten a patient's life. In other words, the daily practice of medicine has always involved decisions that choose alternatives to prolonging patients' lives. The courts are not called upon to participate in these treatment choices. But with the advent of high technology has come the fearsome phrase "pulling the plug," as though tubes and wires and electrical power possess ethical dimensions by themselves. The myth that one must go to court before terminating life support (purveyed even by lawyers themselves, as was so tragically evident in the *Linares* case) is belied by the daily experience of health providers in hospitals, nursing homes and hospices. Efforts at prolonging the life of dying patients are routinely and humanely reduced in favor of palliation, and judicial involvement in these decisions is routinely absent.

Notwithstanding the countless times physicians have terminated life support, there are only about 60 reported cases at the appellate level involving actions by health care professionals to obtain legal permission to terminate life support. And as already noted, although it is impossible to know how many times actions have been brought against physicians in unrecorded lower court cases, not once in this highly litigious country has a physician been found criminally guilty for terminating life support. As one landmark decision acknowledged: "Courts are not the proper place to resolve the agonizing personal problems that underlie these cases. Our legal system cannot replace the more intimate struggle that must be borne by the patient, those caring for the patient, and those who care about the patient."[21]

Finally, we note that even when patients or family members initially insist on treatment, open and honest communication generally limits the risk that a lawsuit will be brought and therefore reduces the need for judicial involvement as a procedural safeguard. When patients and family members already agree, or are eventually persuaded, to withhold or withdraw futile treatment, the legal exposure of health professionals is ever more limited and the appropriateness of obtaining a court ruling is even more doubtful.

Myth Number 8: "Living wills are not legal." By this Meisel refers to the fears of many physicians that if the patient is no longer capable of participating in the process of making treatment decisions personally, all other means of conveying the patient's wishes are legally suspect. Although considerable efforts are now underway to encourage patients to execute "advance directives," namely, documents that specify in writing a patient's wishes or designate a person to act as a proxy decision-maker, these documents are proving to be imperfect solutions to the problem.[22] First of all, perhaps because people find it difficult to contemplate such difficult matters, only a small percentage of patients—even those with life-threatening illness such as metastatic cancer—have executed advance directives.[23] Second, patients turn out to be inconsistent and somewhat unstable in their treatment preferences. Not surprisingly, they change their minds. One obvious explanation for this is that patients (who usually lack a medical education) are rarely fully knowledgeable about treatments and their consequences in advance. If you ask a patient, "Do you want us to get your heart going again if it stops?" almost universally the patient will answer, "Of course." It sounds so easy, why not? (One colleague sardonically suggested that the question might better be phrased: "If you die, do you want us to bring you back to life?") But a patient may arrive at a completely different decision when informed that attempted cardiopulmonary resuscitation could involve forceful, even violent, efforts at compressing the chest cage to the point of fracturing ribs, usually requires thrusting a tube into the trachea and placement on a mechanical ventilator, and often results in outcomes that, in the presence of serious disease like cancer, are rarely successful, and may end with the patient afflicted with serious brain damage. Moreover, even the most fully informed patients facing critical illness may change their minds, and no one, neither patient nor physician, can predict with certainty how a person will feel in the future.

Another, potentially more serious problem with advance directives is that a physician may demand a legal document before acting on a patient's wishes or before withdrawing obviously futile treatment. Our concern in a litigious society is that even though authentic expressions of a patient to a physician or family member or close friend should be sufficient to represent the patient's wishes, such oral or even written statements may be ignored if they are not expressed in "legal" documents. In two states, Missouri and New York, the requirement that there be "clear and convincing" evidence of a patient's treatment wishes has led to judicial travesties. In Chapter 1, we described the agonizing struggle the Cruzan family had to go through to withdraw life support from their permanently unconscious daughter because the state of Missouri would not recognize the authority of her family speaking on her behalf. And as we will describe further in Chapter 8, in New York a relative of a demented and nearly unconscious elderly woman, Mary O'Connor, was prevented from achieving the withdrawal of the patient's feeding tube, because the woman had not specifically predicted her own circumstances. This occurred despite the patient's background as a hospital worker who had repeatedly asked that she not be kept alive in circumstances similar to those of the many patients she had seen. All her previous statements had been discounted by New York's highest court as not fulfilling the "clear and convincing" standard of evidence. In both cases these women were kept alive as much by the law as by medicine.

These cases illustrate therefore that the practice of "defensive medicine" is not always based upon misplaced fears, but is also imposed by unrealistic legal standards. Sadly, though, it is not the physician who suffers the burdens of these unrealistic legal standards so much as the patient.

The problems associated with defensive medicine are not new. When one of the authors was a medical intern in the late 1950s he saw patient after patient admitted to the private service with vague — and usually psychosomatic — abdominal pains who were given what the house staff disparagingly called "the complete radio-opaque work-up" — upper GI series, barium enema, intravenous pyelogram and gall bladder X-ray. A mere few minutes spent with these patients were enough to predict that all the studies would be negative — and the private physician knew they would be. Still, the effort to reassure the patient without performing the ceremony of tests (Doctor, can you be absolutely *sure* there's no cancer in there?) and the fear that lurking behind every complaint was a potential law suit—these were enough to overturn all the lectures of medical school. Today the physician (and the hapless patient) caught up in the quest for fool-proof medicine confront a technology that is even more formidable, involving penetrations and infusions into every recess of the body, and treatments that are in a way far more monstrous even as they are more powerful—hearts and livers from other humans but also from baboons and pigs and even plastic factories, and toxic chemotherapies that render one hairless and marrowless and immunologically helpless, mind-altering drugs and surgeries—the list grows almost daily. And every day the problem becomes more disquieting. As patients continue to expect more from medicine, they look more to the law. They expect medicine to fulfill their hopes and when medicine fails, they somehow expect redress through the courts, as though lawyers and juries can provide what is desired: the miraculous restoration of health and preservation of life.[24] Indeed, only at the very end of life has the law so far acknowledged that perhaps death *is* inevitable. But how long will medicine enjoy even this respite? Understandably we hail—and even more, anticipate—the seemingly endless supply of miracles from modern medicine. But as scientific optimism lurches forward, will the law be far behind?

CHAPTER 7

ETHICAL

IMPLICATIONS

OF MEDICAL

FUTILITY

In the previous chapters we presented an approach to a definition of medical futility against the inevitable background of uncertainty. Realistically, we have to ask: If futility refers to a treatment that doesn't work, how do we *know* it doesn't work? That is, how often should physicians try to achieve a desired medical outcome before they draw conclusions about the success or failure of their efforts? As we pointed out, physicians could try a million times to resuscitate a cadaver and still be vulnerable to the claim that maybe the next time they will succeed. But nowhere in medicine is the physician absolutely certain that a treatment will succeed or fail. Rather, medical practice emerges out of empirical experience, sometimes based on accurate and reliable clinical research, many times, unfortunately, based on hearsay and habit, and false and unreliable claims. Partly because physicians can "never say never," partly because of the seduction of modern technology, and partly out of the misplaced fear of litigation, physicians have shown an increasing tendency to undertake treatments that have no realistic expectation of success. For this reason, we have articulated common-sense criteria for defining medical futility.

We propose that a treatment should be regarded as medically futile if it has not worked in the last 100 cases, or if the treatment fails to restore consciousness or alleviate total dependence on intensive care. This definition provides clear end points and encourages the profession to review data from the past and perform prospective clinical research to determine not only which treatments work but also which treatments do not work. Both kinds of information are essential for doctors and patients to decide when to say yes and when to say no to medical treatments.

In this chapter we consider the ethical implications of our proposal, namely: What should be the obligations of physicians when a treatment has been shown to be medically futile? What should they do and not do? Should physicians be permitted to decide on their own whether or not to offer a futile treatment? Should the medical profession impose on practitioners standards to guide or require compliance? What about patients — how much authority should they have in making such decisions? How much influence should society at large exert upon bedside decisions? What are the possible consequences and risks of granting the power to make futility decisions to any of the above parties? All these questions require an examination of the ethical implications of medical futility — an examination not of definitions but of actions. Seeking the answers inescapably involves us in a reexamination of the very nature of the doctor-patient relationship, particularly of the limits on demands and expectations that can be imposed on doctors.

We begin with the case of Arthur Tanney (not his real name), a 69-year-old man who was admitted for treatment of metastatic carcinoma of the colon. Upon admission to the hospital, he was informed of his rights under the Patient Self-Determination Act to refuse any unwanted treatments. Prior to beginning chemotherapy, Mr. Tanney was informed by Dr. Garland (not her real name) of the anticipated toxicity of the treatment and of the limited chance of good quality and sustained response to treatment. Furthermore, Dr. Garland told Mr. Tanney that in the event of a cardiac arrest during his treatment program, she would not attempt cardiopulmonary resuscitation. She explained that in patients with metastatic cancer, CPR had a negligible chance of success and an almost certain chance of prolonging his suffering before dying in the intensive care unit. In other words, CPR would be futile. Mr. Tanney accepted Dr. Garland's decision and a do not attempt resuscitation (DNAR) order was written. The night after chemotherapy was started, Mr. Tanney developed periods of irregular heartbeat. The physician on duty that night, Dr. Sylvester (also not his real name), rushed to the bedside and, while initiating treatment and arranging immediate transfer to the coronary care unit (CCU), told Mr. Tanney he would attempt CPR if his heart stopped beating effectively. Mr. Tanney nodded in apparent agreement. Shortly thereafter Mr. Tanney underwent a cardiac arrest, and Dr. Sylvester immediately started CPR. These efforts failed, however, and the patient died. The next day at case conference, Dr. Sylvester and Dr. Garland, as well as several other physicians, engaged in heated debate over whether CPR should have been attempted. Dr. Sylvester asserted that it was his personal belief that physicians had a duty to preserve life whenever possible. Dr. Garland countered that a doctor's personal belief should not override a patient's preference. She argued that the patient had previously agreed to a DNAR order. Dr. Sylvester countered that by nodding agreement, the patient had changed his mind.

A conference was arranged and one of us was asked to join the group. During this conference it became apparent that all the physicians were acquainted with a medical journal article that had recently summarized CPR outcomes in several medical centers. The article reported that when CPR was required and attempted in a total of 117 patients with metastatic cancer, not one patient survived to hospital discharge.[1] The author of the report concluded that such treatment was futile and should not be attempted.

The case conference debate then evolved from should CPR have been attempted in Mr. Tanney, to what should physicians do when considering *any* treatment that is likely to fail? In the discussion that followed, several views were aired, including the following: (1) Dr. Sylvester was ethically *permitted* to refrain from attempting CPR but he was also ethically permitted to perform it. In other words, in the presence of a clinical situation in which treatment is futile, it is completely up to the individual physician to act as he or she wishes. (2) Dr. Sylvester should have been *encouraged* not to perform CPR on Mr. Tanney. That is, the findings of the study and the recommendation by the author not to perform CPR might be considered an ethical guideline that physicians are urged but not required to follow. (3) Finally, some argued that once CPR was shown to be futile Dr. Sylvester was ethically *required* as a matter of professional duty to refrain from attempting it.

Several comparisons might prove helpful. In the first instance, allowing Dr. Sylvester to make an individual decision about attempting CPR on a patient with metastatic cancer would be ethically analogous to allowing an ob-gyn physician to decide whether or not to meet a woman's request to perform therapeutic abortion. The medical profession, while accepting abortion as a legal choice for all women, takes an ethically neutral stance and allows individual physicians to refuse to perform the procedure as a matter of personal conscience. Any physician not complying with a patient's request for abortion therefore would not be acting unethically. In the second instance, encouraging, but not requiring, Dr. Sylvester to refrain from attempting CPR is analogous to a physician's decision to support life in patients with permanent vegetative state. Several professional societies have recommended against maintaining patients in permanent vegetative state, yet physicians are not ethically or legally bound to follow these advisory recommendations.[2] Similarly, Dr. Sylvester would be ethically free to attempt CPR in Mr. Tanney; however, refraining from CPR would be regarded as an ethically preferable course. In the third instance, the ethical equivalent is the treatment of patients with human immunodeficiency virus (HIV) infection. The medical profession has specifically mandated that it is the duty of all physicians not to discriminate against patients on the basis of their HIV status. Therefore, a physician who refuses to treat a patient simply because the patient has this condition would violate an ethical duty. Similarly then, attempting CPR in patients with metastatic cancer would be considered *prima facie* wrong for all physicians by virtue of violating professional standards against applying futile treatments to patients. Therefore, this effort was wrong even though Mr. Tanney had requested CPR, because physicians are generally not entitled to breech standards of their profession.

Addressing these three viewpoints provides the central focus for this chapter. In what follows we will proceed stepwise. First, we will argue that physicians are ordinarily *permitted* to refrain from offering or continuing futile treatment. Then we will make the stronger point that physicians should generally be *encouraged* to omit futile therapies. Finally, we will present the still stronger case that physicians should generally be *required* to decline the use of futile interventions. In Chapter 1, we described the historic traditions of medicine that underlie our proposal that medical interventions be regarded as futile where the odds of achieving a medical goal are exceedingly slim or where the quality of outcome to be achieved is exceedingly poor. These same traditions also provide ethical guidance about physicians' responsibilities under futile circumstances. Thus, for example, the well-known Hippocratic Oath identifies the tasks of physicians as twofold: first, to "use treatment to help the sick according to my ability and judgment"; second, "never [to use treatment] with a view to injury and wrongdoing."[3] The oath provides a basis, therefore, for claiming that physicians not only should be *permitted* to refrain from using futile interventions but also should be *encouraged* or *required* to refrain from using futile treatments because such interventions fall outside the scope of helping the sick. Also, they cause "injury and wrongdoing" because they raise false hope, inflict unnecessary pain, prolong suffering, make the dying process less humane and dignified, but most of all because they distract physicians from providing palliation and comfort.

The Platonic tradition gives similar guidance. Medicine is a good so long as "the patient is freed from a great evil, so that it is profitable to submit to the pain and recover health."[4] But a medical regimen is not "a pleasant thing"; patients do not "enjoy it" (261). Plato cautioned that physicians cannot determine whether burdens are offset by benefits by focusing narrowly on specific pathological problems. Instead, the physician must take stock of the whole patient while recognizing that "the part can never be well unless the whole is well." Thus, Plato condemned the physicians of Hellas for "disregarding the whole," and added that "you ought not to attempt to cure the eyes without the head, or the head without the body . . . or the body without the soul" (103). Bringing nutrients to the stomach or breath to the lungs does not necessarily benefit the patient or restore health. Rather, to heal the patient literally means "to make whole or sound in bodily condition." What then should the physician do when wholeness cannot be achieved? What is the physician's ethical duty?

THE WEAKEST ETHICAL STANCE: PHYSICIANS SHOULD BE PERMITTED TO REFRAIN FROM OFFERING FUTILE TREATMENT

A central aim of the profession of medicine is to use the art and science of medicine for the purpose of helping the sick. But futile treatment, by definition, is superfluous to helping the patient. In Mr. Tanney's case, the overwhelming odds were that CPR would not benefit him. It follows then that physicians who refrained from CPR, rather than attempting resuscitation, would in no way be remiss in their duties. Patients who demand nonbeneficial medical treatments from their physicians have an exaggerated and false picture of the duties required of physicians. Moreover, physicians who offer futile interventions deceive their patients and compromise professional standards of medicine. By offering a treatment to a patient, a physician conveys that the treatment represents a medically acceptable alternative. But if the treatment actually is almost certain to fail and the patient is misled into believing in the treatment's efficacy, then the physician has violated the patient's trust. If the physician informs the patient that the treatment is futile and offers it anyway, a confusing double message is thereby conveyed. When physicians prescribe treatments that they are reasonably certain will not improve a patient's condition, they degrade the practice of medicine. They ally medicine with quackery and charlatanism.

The provision of futile treatment is additionally objectionable when the act violates a physician's personal ethical convictions. In this case, a refusal to allow the physician to withhold or withdraw futile interventions does not take seriously the physician's own sense of moral integrity. It would be akin to forcing physicians who oppose abortions to perform them. In these cases, requiring the use of futile interventions wrongly signals that physicians are merely tools for enacting others' (patients', institutions') goals, rather than possessing, as individuals and as members of a profession, independent ethical standards and ends. Thus, we would conclude that at a very minimum physicians should be *permitted* to refrain from offering futile treatment.

A MODERATE ETHICAL STANCE: PHYSICIANS SHOULD BE ENCOURAGED TO REFRAIN FROM OFFERING FUTILE THERAPIES

Suppose that we agree that Dr. Sylvester cannot be compelled to perform CPR on Mr. Tanney. Dr. Sylvester would reasonably conclude, therefore, that he was free either to *use* the futile treatment or to *withhold* it. Either way, his actions would be above reproach.

Some patients and families cling to faith in the miraculous powers of medicine that far exceed medicine's actual scientific capabilities; some hold that they are entitled to their hopes and that medicine is duty-bound to serve them. The difficulty this claim presents is that shocking the heart with high-voltage electricity or pounding on Mr. Tanney's chest in a futile attempt to get the heart started is not an ethically neutral act. Harm is inevitable: ribs can be broken, the trachea damaged by hasty efforts at intubation. Not uncommonly, the brain never completely recovers from oxygen deprivation. In fact, cardiac arrest is the third leading cause of coma, second only to trauma and drug overdose.[5] Most hospitalized patients who undergo CPR never survive to leave the hospital, and some of those who do suffer significant neurological impairment.[6] These harms would be justified only if they were matched by compensatory benefits. But the benefit realized by Mr. Tanney would be only a false hope that he would somehow pull through, that a miracle would happen. The truth is that even if Mr. Tanney had survived the cardiac arrest and retained consciousness, he would only return to the discomfort and suffering associated with his metastatic cancer, and almost certainly would never have survived to hospital discharge. This violates the first ethic of the medical profession: Do no harm.

Even when futile interventions do not exact such a heavy toll, we would argue that physicians should be *encouraged* to withhold and withdraw them because the profession of medicine was never intended to practice non-beneficial medical care. Rather, medicine's aim has always been to help the sick. Affirming this age-old ethic, the President's Commission for the Study of Ethical Problems in Medicine and Biomedical and Behavioral Research stated in 1983 that "the care available from health care professionals is generally limited to what is consistent with role-related professional standards and conscientiously held personal beliefs."[7]

How appropriate is it for medicine to be the only profession with unlimited obligations to the people it serves? Would those who claim that patients and families can demand anything they want from doctors lay similar claims upon other professions? Not at all. Let us look, for example, at the legal profession. A person accused of murder deserves a full and vigorous defense by his attorney. Does that mean that after conviction and life sentence, the permanently incarcerated prisoner can demand that the attorney phone the governor every day in search of a miraculous change of mind and clemency? Surely at some point the lawyer would declare a limit to her professional obligations to the client. A client who orders an architect to design a beautiful but structurally unsound building made of glass would learn that architects are limited by building codes as well as by the codes of their profession. Similarly, physicians are not and never have been obligated to do anything a patient wants, such as treating in expectation of a miracle. Medical treatment is not simply a consumer good to be bought and sold.

Finally, there is an even more important reason why physicians should avoid pursuing futile life-saving treatments. Because the obsessive pursuit of such treatments often causes them to neglect a whole other set of duties — relieving pain and responding to the dying patient's situation in an empathic and caring way. Attention spent on debating useless interventions often distracts physicians from these goals. Indeed, we have found that all too often the medical team is consumed in heated debate over whether or not to attempt aggressive technological interventions, meanwhile giving scant attention to the patient's physical, emotional, and spiritual needs helping the patient achieve as good a death as possible.

A STRONG ETHICAL STANCE: PHYSICIANS SHOULD BE REQUIRED TO REFRAIN FROM OFFERING FUTILE INTERVENTIONS

So far we have defended two progressively stronger claims concerning the ethical responsibilities of physicians in futile circumstances. The weak claim held that physicians are free to withhold or cease futile therapies. The moderate stance maintained that physicians should be encouraged to do so. We now make the still stronger case that physicians should be *required* to forego futile interventions.

The bases for this stronger claim are threefold. First, in the absence of a general professional ethic affirming the scope and limits of physicians' obligations, the meaning and ethical implications of futility are vulnerable to abuse. For example, if Dr. Garland and Dr. Sylvester were free to use "futility" to mean whatever they wish, then their debate over whether to attempt CPR on Mr. Tanney might have had many possible hidden subtexts. Did Dr. Garland think Mr. Tanney too old to be receiving such expensive medical care? Was she subconsciously withholding CPR because the patient was not as pleasant or interesting or grateful as other patients in her care? Perhaps Dr. Sylvester did not experience this, having known Mr. Tanney only briefly. Did Dr. Garland find her time taken away from other patients whom she thought had more need for her and better chances of a successful outcome? All these could lead to the term "futility" being invoked in a variety of subterfuges for rationing, cost containment, or refusals to treat certain categories of patients — HIV-infected or mentally or physically handicapped or elderly individuals. In other words, the absence of a profession-wide standard governing the ethical responsibilities of physicians under futile circumstances invites abuse by allowing physicians to act according to their own (subconscious or deliberately concealed) arbitrary goals. To avoid such abuse, we believe that the profession of medicine must affirm a clear and consistent definition of futility and set systematic standards for its members. Only then can misuses of the term be recognized for what they are. Only then can patients be assured that their wishes and best interests will not be subordinated to inappropriate economic and social considerations.

A second reason for requiring physicians to refrain from futile treatment is that the public rightly looks to the practitioners of medicine to set standards for appropriate medical treatment. Physicians in our society practice medicine as part of a publicly sanctioned profession: society grants the profession authority to certify individual practitioners as competent to act in the best interests of patients. By virtue of receiving such authority, the profession receives the public's trust, just as other professions receive the right and responsibility to provide legal counsel, maintain accounting records, design bridges, and educate. To be worthy of this trust, a profession is obliged to set ethical guidelines for its practitioners. Leaving standards for beneficial and nonbeneficial medical practice to individual clinicians abdicates the medical profession's responsibility to society.

Finally, physicians are ethically obligated to avoid futile medicine because its use exploits the public's fears and feeds inflated ideas about what medicine can achieve. Today not only do Americans fear death, but also those many thousands who made an instant bestseller out of a how-to suicide book published by the Hemlock Society[8] seem to fear *medicine* as an unrestrained force lacking humanity and common sense. Contemporary physicians — even more than did ancient physicians — bear special obligations in this regard because they practice in a society that extols, even worships, technology and clings tenaciously to exaggerated beliefs about what medicine can accomplish. To counter this tendency, the profession of medicine should take a firm and public stand stating the limits of what their profession can and will do. In the absence of such a commitment, individuals and families and society will continue to hold physicians and hospitals hostage by insisting that medicine owes them miraculous feats. Or, they will make rash end-of-life decisions out of distrust for the medical profession, thus depriving themselves of the wide variety of beneficial treatments and care that can be offered.

There are signs that professional medical and biomedical ethical organizations are rising to the challenge of affirming medicine's limits. As early as 1983, the President's Commission for the Study of Ethical Problems in Medicine and Biomedical and Behavioral Research declared: "A health care professional has an obligation to allow a patient to choose from among medically acceptable treatment options . . . or to reject all options. No one, however, has an obligation to provide interventions that would, in his or her judgment, be countertherapeutic."[9] In 1987, the Hastings Center, an internationally recognized bioethics organization, claimed in its *Guidelines on the Termination of Life-Sustaining Treatment and the Care of the Dying* that "if a treatment is clearly futile . . . there is no obligation to provide the treatment."[10]

Other respected medical organizations have begun to follow suit. In 1991, the American Medical Association's Council on Ethical and Judicial Affairs published "Guidelines for the Appropriate Use of Do-Not-Resuscitate Orders." The Council held that CPR may be withheld, even if previously requested by the patient, "when efforts to resuscitate a patient are judged by the treating physician to be futile."[11] In the same year, the American Thoracic Society (an organization of the American Lung Association) took a similar stand, and claimed that "forcing physicians to provide medical interventions that are clearly futile would undermine the ethical integrity of the medical profession."[12] During the same period, the Society of Critical Care Medicine's Task Force on Ethics published a consensus report stating that "treatments that offer no benefit and serve to prolong the dying process should not be employed."[13] More recently the Ethics Committee of the Society of Critical Care Medicine specified severe, irreversible brain damage, irreversible multi-organ failure, and metastatic cancer unresponsive to treatment as categories of "patients who *may* be excluded from the ICU, whether beds are available or not." The Committee also designated "patients who *should* be excluded," as those who refuse intensive care, who are brain-dead, or are in a permanent vegetative state.[14]

OBJECTIONS AND RESPONSES

Why shouldn't the patient, rather than the doctor, always be allowed to decide what to do when treatment is futile? In other words, why should futile treatment not be offered to the patient as an option? Geriatrician Thomas Finucane posed this question in the form of a thought experiment: "If you were to suddenly die now and the probability of surviving with attempted treatment were 1 in 100, would you accept the attempt? Now let us stipulate that the attempt would be free and painless and would, if successful, return you to your current level of function. I would answer 'yes,' promptly. I would answer 'yes' at 1 in 1000. I wouldn't consider the chance to be 'negligible' nor the attempt to be 'inappropriate' in a general sense."[15]

Sure. And if we all had wings we could fly. The problem with formulating the question this way is that in the real world, life-saving medical treatments are never free and painless. Rather, they are by nature invasive, burdensome, and fraught with serious, lingering harms. That is why physicians are expected to use their powers not at will but with care and restraint. However, there is a procedure which meets the criteria of being free, painless, rarely successful, but reputedly now and then miraculous. It is called prayer. The question then becomes: If the patient feels entitled to it, is the *physician* obligated to perform it? We have already argued that physicians are not obligated to offer treatments that are so likely to fail that any success would be considered a miracle. Physicians can offer only what nature allows and cannot accept responsibility for being something they are not—miracle workers. And so, we maintain, physicians are limited in their duty to patients by a common-sense notion of quantitative futility.

We wish also to offer an analogical argument in support of quantitative futility. This argument begins by drawing an analogy between futile treatments and placebos. Placebos (from the word meaning "to please") are medications that display no objective specific activity for the condition being treated. In drug trials involving control subjects, placebos are usually capsules with a small amount of an inert substance like lactose. They are necessary for comparison because the "placebo effect" of a drug, which is perceived as a physiological or psychological benefit and which operates through a psychological mechanism, can be as high as 30 percent or even higher.[16] A dramatic illustration of the placebo effect occurred during World War II when a military pharmacy ran out of narcotics. To the physicians' astonishment, soldiers with severe war injuries, who were not told they were receiving only sterile saline injections, experienced pain relief. What can we conclude from this experience? Even in the case of severe pain, sterile saline might conceivably work. If physicians were morally obligated to offer any treatment that might make a patient feel good or that might conceivably make a patient feel good, the physician would be *obligated,* in the absence of a proven treatment, to offer this placebo. But physicians are *not* morally obligated to offer a placebo when no treatment is available, for good reasons. Any trust between doctor and patient—not to mention the psychological benefits of all medicines—would be destroyed if patients knew that physicians prescribed medicines whether or not they believed in their therapeutic efficacy. Patients would rightly be concerned not only about therapeutic efficacy, but also about therapeutic deception.

But what about qualitative futility? Why shouldn't patients be allowed to decide for themselves the qualities of life they would find acceptable? We believe a distinction is in order. Some qualitatively poor results should indeed be the patient's prerogative. However, other sorts of qualitatively poor results, we believe, fall clearly outside the range of medical goals and need not be offered as options. The clearest of these qualitatively poor results is continued biological life without consciousness. The patient has no right to demand of medicine to be sustained in a state in which he or she has no capacity to appreciate the life prolonged by treatment and no purpose other than mere vegetative survival. The physician should not offer this option or services to achieve it. Other qualitatively poor results include survival that requires the constant monitoring and ventilatory support of the intensive care unit—which effectively prevents the patient from achieving any other life goals, including participation in the human community. Admittedly, seriously ill patients fall along a continuum, and there are well-known examples of the most remark-able achievements of life goals despite the most burdensome handi-caps (the wheelchair-bound theoretical physicist Stephen Hawking comes to mind). However, if survival requires the patient's entire *pre-occupation* with intensive medical treatment, to the extent that the patient cannot achieve any other life goals (thus obviating the goal of medical care), the treatment is producing an effect but not benefit. We believe that it should not be offered to the patient, and the patient's family has no right to demand it.

Specifically excluded from our account is medical treatment for patients for whom such treatment offers the opportunity to achieve life goals, however limited. Thus, patients whose illnesses are severe enough to require frequent hospitalization, patients confined to nurs-ing homes, or patients with severe physical or mental handicaps are not, in themselves, objects of futile treatments. We wish to empha-size: Such patients (or their surrogates) have the right to receive or reject any medical treatment according to their own perception of benefit compared with burdens. We also suggest that the medical profession will respond to our futility proposal not by eagerly seek-ing to give up on severely compromised patients but by looking for better ways to support patients *outside* the intensive care unit—in skilled nursing facilities and even at home, which would permit more interaction between the patient and loved ones and friends and the community at large.

Won't preventing patients from making their own assessment of qualitative futility lead to abuse, neglect, and a retreat to the paternalistic "silent world"[17] *of the past in which doctors avoided communication with their patients? Since physicians are susceptible to abusing power, doesn't granting the health pro-fessions authority to limit futile treatment grant too much authority?* We acknowledge that the potential for abuse is present and share this concern and would deplore the use of our proposal to excuse doctors from engaging patients in ongoing informed dialogue. But we be-lieve that by holding physicians to openly declared standards of med-ical futility, our proposal not only authorizes physicians to exercise professional judgment but also limits their power and prevents the arbitrary exercise of ethically indefensible actions. And we must point out that the alternative—allowing patients unlimited demands—is also subject to abuse, for example, when patients and surrogates intimidate hospitals into providing extravagant, nonbeneficial care by threatening to sensationalize their case in the media.

Isn't the determination of medical futility purely a value judgment that physicians are no better equipped than lay people to render? We agree that physicians could never claim authority to render futility judgments under the guise of some purely objective and value-free "scientific" or "technical" expertise. Instead, the proper basis for assigning physicians authority to set standards for the practice of medicine is that an ethical dimension is an integral component of the historical and contemporary role of the profession in society. As the philosopher and medical ethicist Margaret Battin astutely observes, even when the patient gives informed consent to treatment, "it is the physician who identifies the problem, frames any suggested solution to it, and controls how many alternative solutions are proposed. The patient cannot know whether the problem could be seen in some other way or as some different sort of problem, whether other sorts of solutions could be proposed, whether in making the choice to give or withhold consent he or she is making a choice among all the reasonable alternatives, and, sometimes, whether there is really any problem at all."[18] Thus it is clear that in almost every conceivable circumstance, physicians wield enormous power in modern society, and for this reason society rightly expects them to show restraint, and to practice their craft in an ethical way. The fact that society deplores those who practice medicine solely in order to make a profit, achieve status, or selfishly exploit their power, reveals that we hold physicians to a high moral standard and expect them to use their skills to help sick people and promote the good of society. This expectation will continue to be justified only so long as the profession of medicine espouses and practices according to ideals of service and advocacy for patients.

It should also be emphasized again, however, that physicians are obligated to make *medical* decisions, namely decisions aimed at healing the suffering patient. Preserving biologic existence is not one of those decisions. Vitalist notions that a permanently unconscious body or a dead body whose heart and lungs are being kept active by mechanical means — that these conditions must be prolonged — are not medical concepts. And although some members of society may hold such imperatives as deeply felt beliefs, they cannot be imposed on health professionals any more than a deep belief in the importance of teaching Creationism can be imposed on the educational profession.

Won't requiring physicians to refrain from using futile treatments unfairly violate the religious convictions of some patients, and even of some doctors and nurses? This is an important question, since most persons in this country — including patients and health professionals — either observe or are significantly influenced by religious beliefs. Nurses are peculiarly vulnerable in these situations. Following their own religious beliefs, patients can demand and refuse treatments, and physicians can order and refuse to order them. But nurses by the nature of their intermediary role in the medical hierarchy — obligated to both parties — are often locked in the middle of painful conflicts. Their power to control events, not to mention their own actions, is severely limited and their sense of job security often threatened. Indeed, some of the most difficult ethical consultations we have conducted deal with the so-called "moral stresses" of nurses forced to carry out orders that they feel are harmful and inappropriate.

However, as the theologian James W. Walters points out, religion offers "fundamental perspectives which inform society's dilemmas," but, like other forces in society, religion "must make a public case for its views."[19] And contrary to the notion of a single immutable theology, in fact all religious traditions have undergone re-examination and re-interpretation throughout history, even within the Catholic Church, which is traditionally regarded as representing timeless unchanging views. Catholic scholar and jurist John T. Noonan Jr. writes:

> Wide shifts in the teaching of moral duties, once presented as part of Christian doctrine by the magisterium, have occurred. In each case one can see the displacement of a principle or principles that had been taken as dispositive — in the case of usury, that a loan confers no right to profit; in the case of marriage, that all marriages are indissoluble; in the case of slavery, that war gives a right to enslave and that ownership of a slave gives title to the slave's offspring; in the case of religious liberty, that error has no rights and the fidelity to the Christian faith may

be physically enforced. . . . In the course of this displacement of one set of principles, what was forbidden became lawful (the cases of usury and marriage); what was permissible became unlawful (the case of slavery); and what was required became forbidden (the persecution of heretics).[20]

Professor Charles Curran also objects to a Roman Catholic theology that presents itself as immutable, eternal, and unchanging, rather than emphasizing "evolution, growth, change and historicity."[21] And the Catholic theologian Richard McBrien of Notre Dame agrees that "there are many different approaches to theological issues." These approaches are inevitably influenced by historical context and evolving contingencies that require repeated interpretations with respect to the specific application of religious principles to the ever-changing complexities of modern medicine. "All the principles that the church lives by," McBrien declares, "are principles that come out of its own experience."[22]

In the past, Bible-quoting religious leaders have used religious principles to justify slavery and suppression of women, to name just two examples of values almost universally rejected today by mainstream American theologians and society. It is particularly important to keep this in mind with regard to the medical context. Both the Jewish and Christian traditions make the claim that life is of supreme value, a gift of God to be held in trust. But what exactly is meant by life? Biological existence? Cells possessing human chromosomes? Personhood? As we have already noted, modern medical technology has created many states of life between health and death that were unimaginable in the days when the major religions evolved.

In the best of circumstances, physicians and members of the clergy pool their skills and knowledge to help patients come to terms with their situation. Sometimes hospital chaplains can play a particularly valuable and comforting role by correcting a devout family's misapprehensions about what is ordained in their religion. For example, Catholicism does *not* absolutely forbid the use of pain medications that might accelerate death, nor forbid the withdrawal of life support under any circumstances. In fact, under the principle of "double effect," it is Catholic theology that has provided the most cogent moral guidance in the first instance, namely that as long as the physician's intent is to achieve a good (alleviating suffering) then an unavoidable side-effect (increasing the risk of death) is not deemed sinful. In the second instance, Catholicism does not require physicians to impose on their patients "extraordinary" treatments, namely interventions that are capable of achieving little or no benefit or whose burdens outweigh any benefits.

One example of a thoughtful and knowledgeable interpretation of essential religious values in the light of modern medical technology is provided by the Christian physician, James Reitman, citing Eccles. 9:3–6 (*New International Version*):

> This is the evil in everything that happens under the sun: The same destiny overtakes all. The hearts of men, moreover, are full of evil and there is madness in their hearts while they live, and afterward they join the dead. Anyone who is among the living has hope—even a live dog is better off than a dead lion!
> For the living know that they will die,
> but the dead know nothing;
> they have no further reward,
> and even the memory of them is forgotten.
> Their love, their hate
> and their jealousy have long since vanished;
> never again will they have a part
> in anything that happens under the sun.[23]

Reitman found in these biblical lines the fundamental wisdom that death is impartial and inevitable for all, that the motivation of human beings is impure and their insight is lacking. Nevertheless, the passage points out, life has meaning (which justifies hope), regardless of status, as long as life exists. But what gives meaning to life is the exercise of awareness ("For the living *know* that they will die"); emotive responsivity ("Their love, their hate and their jealousy"); and volitional capacity (having "a part in anything that happens under the sun.") Reitman argues that as the capacity for any or all of these qualities erodes with illness and suffering, there is a progressive decrease in the potential for meaning and hope. Physicians should take into account on an ongoing basis this eroding potential in making medical decisions, including providing aggressive life support or withholding such treatments on grounds of futility. The duty of the physician, he states, is not to err in either direction, *"either of usurping the prerogative of a sovereign God over life [as defined in the Ecclesiastes] or of prematurely removing hope."*[24]

With regard to medical treatments, Catholic moralists have long distinguished between ordinary (obligatory) and extraordinary (non-obligatory) measures. In the Catholic tradition, futile or nonbeneficial treatments as well as extremely burdensome treatments, are not held to be obligatory. Thus, although life preservation is regarded as a value requiring ordinary efforts, it is not a paramount or overriding value requiring extraordinary efforts.

In the Jewish tradition, the commentary of the fourteenth-century Provençal Halakhist R. Menahem ha-Meiri is often cited today as one of the authorities for the mandate to pursue maximal efforts at life preservation: "Even if [a person found alive under a fallen house] cannot live more than an hour, in that hour he may repent and utter the confession."[25] Clearly, the commentary emerged from a time when human biological existence and personhood were experienced as coterminous, with consciousness typically ending only a short time before death. Such reasoning did not anticipate or take into account the impossibility of confession during the decades of unconsciousness possible in a patient preserved by modern technology in the permanent vegetative state. As the contemporary Jewish theologian Rabbi Immanuel Jakobovits points out, all the authoritative Jewish sources refer to an individual in whom death is expected to be imminent, "three days or less in rabbinic references" (263). It is also interesting to note that rabbinical distinctions were made between acts viewed as hastening death, such as closing the eyes of the dying person, and acts considered "impediments to death" (263), such as the noise made by a nearby woodchopper or salt placed on the tongue. Thus, though they come from a historical context that no longer exists, these theological pronouncements nevertheless resonate with our own modern debate about the use of technologies and food and fluids that "prolong dying." Dr. Fred Rosner and Rabbi J. David Bleich ask, "Yet who can make the fine distinction between prolonging life and prolonging the act of dying? The former comes within the physician's reference, the latter does not"(264). Indeed, the sources for Jewish ethics, namely the Talmud, Torah, and rabbinical commentaries, reveal a rich history of interpretation in each era and society, activities that continue today.[26] As the Catholic scholar John Noonan summarizes: "In new conditions, with new insight, an old rule need not be preserved in order to honor a past discipline."[27]

It should be evident, therefore, that medicine cannot assume that religion imposes fixed and detailed rules on what constitutes futile treatment and whether or not to attempt them. Furthermore, in our society, the separation of church and state both protects religious diversity and restrains any group from imposing a single theological interpretation on public policy formation. Under the Constitution, every citizen of this country is free to hold any religious conviction, but the state is not permitted to impose that conviction on other individuals or on society in general. Similarly, standards of medical treatment cannot reflect the religious creed of any single group, but instead should represent the outcome of open and reasoned debate encompassing a wide range of religious and other values. Only in this manner does the profession receive the sanction of the entire society that it is called upon to serve. And although particular individuals and groups in this country can always be expected to make claims on medicine that are based on religious and other grounds, the profession of medicine is rightly governed by values and standards that are its own. One compromise our country has chosen to allow for religious pluralism and prevent imposition of religious beliefs on others has been to enable those with specific religious convictions to form their own health care systems. One example is Catholic hospitals that do not perform abortions. In like manner, religious groups who demand medical treatments outside the mainstream of society, such as unlimited life-support for patients in permanent vegetative state, could develop their own health care facilities devoted to treating members who share this belief.[28]

Won't granting the medical profession authority to define medical futility and set ethical standards start us down a perilous and slippery slope, returning us to the unhappy days of physician paternalism or, worse, to a society and medical profession that contributed to the horrors of the Nazi era? How can we be assured that physicians won't apply racial and other invidious stereotypes when evaluating patients' quality of life? How can we be confident that physicians won't extend their authority from extreme cases, in which interventions are clearly futile, to other kinds of cases where the quality of life associated with an intervention is impaired, but remains well worth living? How can we be assured that physicians granted the authority to withdraw futile treatments will not proceed to take it on themselves to actively hasten their patients' deaths? In short, what will stop physicians who withhold and withdraw life support from persons in a persistent vegetative state today from tomorrow withholding treatments from or arbitrarily killing persons because they are elderly or have mental or physical disabilities? We do not dismiss such concerns lightly. The abuse of futility can produce devastating consequences, and physicians are not immune from prejudices and stereotypes legion in the larger society. Nonetheless, we reiterate our belief that the best way to stem possible abuses is to make policies that are explicit and public regarding the definition and ethical implications of medical futility. Most important, and a crucial distinction from the attitudes of the Nazi era, decisions about medical futility must be patient-centered and not grounded in some ideology or notion of societal good. And to those who fear the potential abuses of medical futility we must sadly report our everyday experiences. Today, every day, at the bedside, futility judgments are being made in a variety of inconsistent ways. And the physicians making these judgments are not accountable to their colleagues or to the public, nor are their judgments measured against specific and openly declared professional standards. By demanding that physicians be held to such standards, we actually *limit* the power of physicians to impose their will.

Isn't all this talk about futility in reality nothing more than a convenient code for talking about rationing and cost-containment? If so, isn't it manipulative and unethical to disguise economic matters in this fashion? We respond by pointing out (as we did Chapter 5) that rationing, cost-containment, and futility have very different meanings and ethical implications. That is why it is essential for us to address these issues openly. Failure to do so will continue the confusion and emotional distortions that have made sensible discourse so difficult and subject to political posturing. Futility refers to a specific treatment-benefit relationship in a particular patient. Futility means that a treatment offers no reasonable benefit to that patient—whether or not it is cheap or easily available. In contrast, rationing refers to treatments that *do* offer benefits but that cannot be offered because they are too costly or scarce or because other patients have been given priority of access. Cost-containment also differs in its meaning and ethical implications from futility in that the goal of cost-containment is to reduce overall medical expenditures.

Sometimes, as we have already pointed out, the question of providing medical treatment is posed in terms of economics alone. "If I am rich [the question may go] and can afford to pay for years of intensive medical treatment for my child's permanent vegetative state, why can't I have it?" Our answer is: "Because you really *can't* afford to pay for it. Because the cost is not merely the room rate of the ICU and the various supplies and professional fees, but rather involves a fraction of a far more vast sum of money (taken from taxing others), including that expended on constructing the hospital facilities, on developing the treatments, on the training all the people who have provided every aspect of health care, and on the research and training of all those who trained them, and so on. But most of all, you can't pay for the health care taken away from others while it is being provided for your child." So our response to those who call for the freedom to have any medical care they want is that in the process of health care reform, our democratic society first must provide a "decent minimum" satisfactory to the society as a whole. Beyond that decent minimum our society will certainly allow "buy-ups" for those who wish to seek additional medical goals, such as cosmetic surgery, perhaps. But it does not follow, therefore, that persons will be entitled to buy *anything* they want from health providers, even treatments that serve no medical goal.

CONCLUSION

In closing, we submit that physicians should generally be required to refrain from using futile interventions. This general ethical stance should be publicly endorsed by the medical profession, embodied in institutional policies, and presented clearly and frankly to the public. Such a stance includes a candid acknowledgment that doctors cannot arrogantly offer nor patients unreasonably demand unlimited treatments. It forces us to re-examine the doctor-patient relationship in this era of modern medicine. In the absence of a clear and consistent ethical standard, choices will continue to be made regarding the use of futile therapies, but they will be subject to various abuses. These less-visible approaches may give comfort to those who do not wish to admit or deal with what is already occurring. Yet critics should recognize that, in the final analysis, covert tactics are a more convenient way to dispose of unwanted persons than are openly acknowledged definitions and standards. Explicitly stated criteria and values hold out the promise of evolving toward a more ethical system of health care, which is in the interest of patients as well as physicians.

CHAPTER 8

THE WAY IT

IS NOW / THE

WAY IT OUGHT

TO BE: FOR

PATIENTS

THE WAY IT IS NOW

The case of Mary O'Connor, a 77-year old widow who suffered a series of progressively debilitating strokes that left her bedridden, demented, and paralyzed, is often cited in ethics and the law as an important case in the evolving debate over the right of family members to refuse unwanted treatment on behalf of patients. It also provides us with unexpected insights into the debate over medical futility.

The case entered the courts in 1988, when Mrs. O'Connor's inability to swallow led her doctor at the Westchester County Medical Center to order a nasogastric feeding tube. Her two daughters objected, claiming that such treatment was against their mother's previously and repeatedly expressed wishes that she not be maintained on artificial life support. The New York Court of Appeals, after reviewing the evidence considered by the lower court, concluded that it was not "clear and convincing" that Mrs. O'Connor really knew what she was talking about, despite her background of twenty years working at Jacobi Hospital and confronting severely ill patients on a daily basis; despite the experience of nursing her husband's stepmother, father, and two brothers through long illnesses before they died; and despite the woman's own experience with hospitalization for congestive heart failure. "There is nothing," the majority concluded, "other than speculation to persuade the factfinder that her expressions were more than an immediate reaction to the unsettling experience of seeing or hearing of another's unnecessarily prolonged death."[1]

Judge Simons wrote a scathing dissenting opinion, and it is instructive to view the battle that took place between him and Chief Judge Wachtler, who wrote the majority opinion.

Both judges acknowledged that Mrs. O'Connor was incapable of expressing her treatment wishes because of severe brain damage.

Yet, Judge Wachtler concluded that she should receive feedings through a gastric tube because "death from starvation and especially thirst was a painful way to die and . . . Mrs. O'Connor would, therefore, experience extreme, intense discomfort since she is conscious, alert, capable of feeling pain and sensitive to even mild discomfort."

In his dissent Judge Simons attacked the very basis for ignoring Mrs. O'Connor's stated wishes on the grounds that they were not "clear and convincing." For who *could* meet such evidentiary standards if a woman with many years of life and considerable experience with illness and health care could not? Mrs. O'Connor had repeatedly expressed her values "in the only terms familiar to her, and she expressed them as clearly as a layperson should be asked to express them, and found 'monstrous' the imposition of artificial means to maintain her under these circumstances."

Simons apparently lacked sufficient medical knowledge to reject Judge Wachtler's most glaring misrepresentation, the use of emotionally stereotyped words such as *thirst* and *starvation,* which fail to take into account that dying patients often experience more distress if food and fluids are forced upon them, and which can be alleviated in any case by good medical practice and humane care, including pain medications and sedatives.[2] However, he did draw attention to discrepancies between the testimony accepted by the trial court and the distorted descriptions of the patient by Judge Wachtler:

> Preliminarily, it is important to clearly understand the facts of Mary O'Connor's condition. Mrs. O'Connor is a 77-year-old widow who has suffered a series of progressively debilitating strokes that have left her bedridden, substantially paralyzed and incapable to care for herself. . . . She is neither comatose nor in a vegetative state, but she responds only sporadically to simple questions or commands and then frequently inappropriately. The doctors agree that the neurological damage from the stroke is irreparable and no hope exists for significant improvement in her mental or physical condition. . . . Both daughters testified that since their mother was hospitalized at the medical center, they have visited her daily, sometimes twice a day and, despite their efforts to detect some sign of consciousness, their Mother has never spoken or responded to them in any way even by facial expression or hand movement. . . . This evidence was accepted by the trial court and the Appellate Division and under rules of law too well known to require citation, it binds this court. Nevertheless, the majority [meaning

Judge Wachtler's written opinion] characterizes Mrs. O'Connor's condition in quite different terms stating: "She is awake and conscious; she can feel pain, responds to simple commands, can carry on limited conversations, and is not experiencing any pain. She is simply an elderly person who as a result of several strokes suffers certain disabilities, including an inability to feed herself or eat in a normal manner."[3]

Judge Simons points out that no reliable witness described Mrs. O'Connor as "conscious" or "alert." He argues that her inability to swallow is

a substantial loss of a bodily function, analogous to a patient's loss of kidney function requiring dialysis to sustain life or the inability to breathe without the aid of a respirator. Indeed, Mrs. O'Connor cannot even ask to be fed because . . . she could not comprehend that question. . . . While she may not be terminally ill in the sense that death is imminent, she is dying because she has suffered severe injuries to her brain and body, which, if nature takes its course, will result in death. Full medical intervention will not cure or improve her, it will only maintain her in a rudimentary state of existence.[4]

Particularly noteworthy is how Judge Simons ventured beyond mere dissent to invoke a powerful phrase: *a rudimentary state of existence*. It seems evident to us that the judge was attempting to grant recognition not only to the values of Mrs. O'Connor as communicated to her daughters but also to a fundamental value of society, a value that in fact both sides are claiming to represent, one that often is described in abstract terms as "respect for life" or "sanctity of life."[5] The principal is explicitly or implicitly invoked in every abortion and euthanasia debate. At best it expresses itself in the cautionary query: What safeguards are necessary to prevent the debasement of human life? At worst it shuts off discussion with clamorous references to the Holocaust. Conservatives invoke this principle when they claim that even if a developing fetus is not yet conscious and does not yet have interests of its own, it is nonetheless valuable and merits our dignity and respect. Many conservatives make a parallel claim at the end of life: Even if a human being is in permanent vegetative state and ceases forever to be a person with interests and rights, human life itself is precious and worth preserving.

One problem with the "sanctity of life" principle is that it is often put forward as an ethical absolute that allows for no further ethical dialogue. Properly understood, however, the principle leaves wide open the question of what constitutes showing "proper respect" for human life. In the case of abortion, for example, it is possible to accept the idea that human life is intrinsically valuable while at the same time holding that human life has greater intrinsic value the more fully formed it is, so that a late abortion is more morally troublesome than an early one is. Or someone might endorse the "sanctity of life" principle, yet interpret it as forbidding bringing into existence a human being that will not be properly nurtured and cared for. We submit that the "sanctity of life" principle in fact raises more questions than it answers.

But the "sanctity of life" issue does introduce the inescapable question: Is it possible to honor the wishes of patients like Mrs. O'Connor without plummeting down the slippery slope to a new Nazi era? And one wonders: Does this lurk in the shadow of Judge Wachtler's opinion? And is this the fear that Judge Simons is trying to clear away from the debate?

It is perhaps revealing that Judge Wachtler had to misrepresent the clinical condition of Mrs. O'Connor to claim to protect her "sanctity of life" *against* any evidence of her wishes. In contrast, Judge Simons accepted both the trial court's description of her clinical condition and the testimony of her wishes as being *most consistent with* protecting her "sanctity of life." For, as Judge Simons may have been well aware, Mrs. O'Connor is not alone. Survey after survey has made clear the universality of Mrs. O'Connor's view that it would be "monstrous" to be maintained by medicine in a "rudimentary state of existence." This attitude is shared by every major religious group: 79 percent of Catholics, 70 percent of Jews, and 75 percent of Protestants favor allowing withdrawal of life support from a hopelessly ill or irreversibly unconscious patient. And polls have consistently shown that a high percentage (76 percent) of Americans believe that the law should sanction the withdrawal of life-sustaining treatment (including nutrition and hydration) from hopelessly ill or irreversibly comatose patients if they or their family request it.[6] Exceptions in which demands have been made to keep an unconscious or barely conscious life going by artificial means are rare. And as we discussed in Chapter 4, although such demands may be guided by sincere religious beliefs, even so it is hard for families to separate their own emotional and financial considerations from the patient's best interests.

In his dissent, Judge Simons noted regretfully:

> In simpler times, decisions involving life and death were made by the family and its advisers based upon the patient's wishes or what the family thought best as justified by its knowledge of the patient's values and its sense of what the patient's best interests required. In today's world, the sick are removed to hospitals where a broad array of mechanical equipment awaits, capable of prolonging life even though no cure or repair is possible. Necessarily, others must be involved in this decision whether to use it. . . . Few, if any, patients can meet the demanding standard the majority has adopted and the requirements of precision will necessarily be satisfied by pragmatic judicial decisions of what is "best" under the circumstances. . . . The majority disguising its action as an application of the rule in self-determination, has made its own substituted judgment by improperly finding facts and drawing inferences contrary to the facts found by the courts below. Judges, the persons least qualified by training, experience or affinity to reject the patient's instructions, have overridden Mrs. O'Connor's wishes, negated her long-held values on life and death, and imposed on her and her family their ideas of what her best interest requires.[7]

In the end, society must adjudicate the debate between Judge Wachtler and Judge Simons: What level of human existence is medicine obligated to prolong? For in deciding whether the 77-year-old widow knew what she was talking about, we are deciding what are the underlying assumptions of society. Were her statements so consistent with "long-held values on life and death" by society at large that they could be accepted as clear and convincing evidence? Or were her statements so out of keeping with general societal values that they had to be viewed with extreme suspicion? Here is where the public enters the futility debate.

In previous chapters, we have made the case that health providers should not pursue treatments that offer no reasonable chance of benefiting the patient. We have argued that physicians have no obligation to provide such futile treatments, even if demanded. Indeed, we have argued that physicians have a positive obligation to say no. Although medicine has great powers, it does not have unlimited powers, and although medicine has great obligations, it does not have unlimited obligations. The duty of the profession is to benefit the patient. Nothing less and nothing more.

In this chapter we turn for the first time to the role that patients and society at large might play in defining the obligations and limits of medicine and the associated standards of medical futility. How can society possibly undertake this task? Is it possible to reach any consensus at all about this contentious issue? The philosopher Daniel Callahan doubts this possibility, stating that there is "no political process to allow physicians and lay people together to develop appropriate standards [for medical futility]."[8] Although it is unclear what kind of "political process" Callahan has in mind, he could not realistically expect physicians and society at large to unite spontaneously in a generally accepted definition. Nor, in our opinion, is the well-known process for establishing rationing priorities through town meetings, that took place in Oregon, readily adaptable to defining futility. Nevertheless the political process must begin.

Public opinion researcher Daniel Yankelovich points out that in a participatory democracy, it is possible to achieve over time what he calls "public judgment," namely a particular form of public opinion that exhibits "(1) more thoughtfulness, more weighing of alternatives, more genuine engagement with an issue, more taking into account a wide variety of factors than ordinary public opinion as measured in opinion polls, and (2) more emphasis on the normative, valuing, ethical side of questions than on the factual, informational side."[9]

Yankelovich cites several examples of public opinion in which people appear to understand the consequences of their views and have formed relatively stable and consistent judgments. One example is the death penalty. Public polls reveal that since the mid-1960s, more and more people in our country have supported the death penalty, reaching an average of 73 percent favoring the death penalty for murder and other serious crimes in the late 1980s. Interviews with those who support the death penalty reveal that they have struggled with the question, and are aware of its implications. They recognize, for example, that one implication of instituting a death penalty is that some innocent people will die. Knowing this does not cause them to change their mind. The public also discriminates between different circumstances in which the death penalty may be imposed, with fewer people supporting capital punishment for crimes committed by minors or by mentally retarded persons.

In the area of abortion, public opinion has also remained relatively stable over the last fifteen years, and the public makes various ethical distinctions. A 1989 poll suggests that 49 percent believe that abortion should be legal, 39 percent add critical qualifications, and 9 percent believe that abortion should not be permitted under any circumstances. Yankelovich concludes that

> support for abortion when the pregnancy threatens the mother's life has remained steady for years at about the 85 percent level, and at about the 75–85 percent level "if there is a strong chance of a serious defect in the baby" or in the case of pregnancy resulting from rape. The public is more closely divided over the right to abortion when "the family has a very low income and cannot afford any more children" . . . or when "a married woman does not want to have any more children" . . . Opposition to abortion reached majority status (about 60 percent) in response to questions probing views on abortion for women who seem to lack a concrete or compelling reason for ending their pregnancy.[10]

Yankelovich likens the gradual coming to a public judgment to a biological process.[11] It begins with dawning awareness of an issue, moves to a sense of urgency and discovery of choices, through wishful thinking, to a more mature stage of taking a stand intellectually and integrating this stand with moral and emotional judgments. When public consensus develops in this manner, and when it reflects "open, inclusive moral discovery and growth,"[12] it solidifies a sense of common purpose and carries moral force in the community.

Yankelovich distinguishes three crucial stages in the evolution of public judgment. The first consists of consciousness raising: the public learns about an issue and becomes aware of its existence and meaning. A second stage in the evolution of public judgment is working through. Working through begins after consciousness has been raised and individuals begin to face the needs for change. In the case of medical futility, change must involve altering attitudes and expectations, as well as overt behavior. It will require society to change widely held expectations about what medicine and science can accomplish. A third stage in the evolution of public judgment is resolution. Resolution is multifaceted and occurs at cognitive, emotional, and moral levels. Cognitive resolution requires people to "clarify fuzzy thinking, reconcile inconsistencies, break down the walls of artificial compartmentalizing that keep them from recognizing related aspects of the same issue, take relevant facts and new realities into account, and grasp the consequences of various choices with which they are presented."[13] Emotional resolution "means that people have to confront their own ambivalent feelings, accommodate themselves to unwelcome realities and overcome their urge to procrastinate and to avoid the issue."[14] Moral resolution involves struggling to do the right thing, even when this requires setting aside one's own needs and desires.

THE WAY IT OUGHT TO BE

We have already argued that the health professions must initiate the futility debate because they have received the public trust to define and act in accordance with standards of beneficence. That is, the definition of medical futility must be consistent with the primary goal of medicine, which is to benefit patients. This goal involves limits as well as obligations. Indeed, in Chapter 5 we pointed out how important it is to separate issues of futility from rationing in order that doctors not be regarded as prostitutes willing to do anything for money. Yet the fact that health professionals are given the authority to define standards of medical practice does not imply that society has no role in this area or must passively accept whatever they decide.[15] To the contrary, society is the final arbiter of whether the performance of health professionals helps people and benefits society. Where this does not occur, society exercises its role in changing professional behavior by regulating the professions, passing laws to govern professional conduct, or otherwise exerting an influence to alter professional conduct. For example, if physicians were to announce that it is consistent with professional standards to offer aid-in-dying (voluntary euthanasia or assisted suicide) to terminally ill patients who request it, society would ultimately decide whether these acts are permissible in terms of benefitting patients. To express its will, society would most likely act by lobbying state representatives to pass laws that either permitted or prohibited this practice, or by electing representatives who supported such laws. The U.S. Supreme Court would serve as the final judge of whether such laws were valid and constitutional.

With respect to medical futility, health professionals have begun to debate futility's definition and ethical implications. We have already noted that medical organizations (such as the American Medical Association, the American Heart Association, the Society of Critical Care Medicine, and the American Thoracic Society) and health care facilities are beginning to recognize medical futility explicitly and clarify health professionals' responsibilities in this area.

In every case, however, the determination that a particular intervention is futile transcends empirical medical knowledge. For in every case the term *futility* is applied, we either predict that the chance of a significant benefit occurring is so slim that it is futile, or we judge that the qualitative outcome will be so exceedingly poor as to be futile. Yet, as skeptics point out, nothing in physicians' and nurses' medical training prepares them to become experts about ethical matters. Nothing in the study of science teaches a person to know what quality of outcome is worthwhile and what chance of benefit is worth taking. In the domain of ethics, we must assume that health professionals are no better equipped than the next person. If this is correct, why doesn't it follow that health professionals should have no greater authority than patients to assess the ethical aspect of medical futility? Why should not health professionals simply tell their patients what the effects of a particular intervention are likely to be and invite patients to judge for themselves whether those effects count as significant benefits or not? In other words, why shouldn't patients, rather than health professionals, decide the ends of medicine?

We have addressed this question to some extent in Chapter 7, yet at this point we need to explain more fully what role patients should play and why. We begin by noting that medical futility is hardly the only area where medical decisions have ethical components. Value decisions are an ever-present part of the practice of medicine. However, the role of any particular doctor or nurse in setting ethical standards is limited, because each is held to standards of the entire medical or nursing profession. The profession as a whole, rather than the individual provider at the bedside, determines the ethical values and purposes of medicine.

Acknowledging that the authority of health professionals to

practice medicine and to establish standards of medical care is granted by society suggests that medicine's authority cannot be absolute. Indeed, it always remains contingent upon society continuing to grant its approval. Ultimately, the profession must receive society's sanction to continue to receive the public's trust. If health professionals cease to act for the good of their patients and the society, then their authority will and should be limited. For instance, when the public suspects that physicians are not serving as advocates but are instead promoting their own welfare at the public's expense, medical authority is restricted. This happened most recently when studies showed that physicians who owned their own laboratories and X-ray facilities ordered significantly more tests on their patients than physicians who did not stand to gain from these profit-making facilities. The public was appropriately outraged at what it regarded as physicians putting their own financial interests ahead of their patients' best interests, and the government intervened and regulated physician ownership.

As the health professions begin to reach a consensus about the meaning of medical futility, members of society should evaluate this consensus and decide whether it is acceptable to them. Physicians and other health professionals can assist the public in reaching cognitive, emotional, and moral resolution by taking the initiative in clearly pointing out the alternatives and the consequences different alternatives. The options we have presented throughout the book are two-fold. One option is for society to require health professionals to offer patients treatments that are unlikely to provide significant benefits. As a consequence of this approach, doctors and nurses would be forced to narrow their understanding of their professional responsibilities and see the ends of medicine and health care simply as executing patients' wishes, rather than benefiting them. Requiring health professionals to provide futile treatment means also that society must be willing to underwrite the costs of nonbeneficial treatments and spend larger and larger amounts of money on health care.

A second option is for society to assign to health professions the primary responsibility of setting ethical standards in this area. This means asking doctors and nurses to renew their commitment to helping patients. Although patients remain free to decide among medically viable options, health professionals would determine what these options include. Authorizing health professionals to limit the use of medically futile treatments also means that society is unwilling to pay the high cost of applying marginally beneficial technologies, and is determined instead to invest limited health care dollars in areas where they are of greater benefit.

We close this chapter by issuing a call to action to patients. According to Yankelovich, a successful call to action must include these elements: a vision of what the hoped-for future will look like, specific goals to pursue in reaching that future, strategies for achieving those goals, and techniques for implementing strategies.

1. A Vision. Our vision of health care is patient-centered.[16] It pictures the ends of medicine to include healing the sick and helping and caring for persons. These goals cannot be met by treatments that merely produce physiological effects on an organ system or body part. Instead, medical treatments must provide therapeutic benefits to persons. Keeping a heart beating or lungs breathing does not accomplish medicine's goals when a person will never regain consciousness, or never leave the intensive care unit, or never be free from intense and unremitting pain. A patient-centered approach regards the subject of medical care to be the suffering person, not the biological organism or failing body part. Specifically, the public must speak out against court decisions that order anencephalic newborns and patients in permanent vegetative state to be kept alive by medical technology if the public does not want to end up being treated in ghoulish versions of the Frankenstein Medical Center.

2. Specific Goals to Pursue. The most important goal is for patients and the public to insist that health professionals reaffirm their commitment to benefit patients. As we have noted, evidence suggests that the phenomenon of overtreating patients and acting contrary to conscience is widespread among health professionals, with nearly half (46 percent) of physicians and nurses at five hospitals reporting acting against their conscience in providing treatment to critically and terminally ill patients.[17] Patients should no longer tolerate this or accept the high toll it exacts on individuals and families.

Reaffirming a commitment to benefit the patient is an avowal of the oldest ethical traditions of medicine, expressed most eloquently in the Hippocratic writings. As we described in Chapter 1, Hippocratic medicine teaches that medicine's goal is healing the sick and this is accomplished through assisting and working with nature. According to Hippocratic ethics, medicine is *techne,* which implies doing. In doing, one is "bound . . . by the potentialities of the object . . . [and] by those of the *techne* itself."[18]

A second goal that can help to make our vision a reality is for society to insist that health professions conduct and publish empirical research regarding the outcomes of medical treatments on different patient groups, including both positive outcomes (to be achieved) and negative outcomes (to be avoided). Ultimately, knowledge about the outcomes of medical treatments can provide the empirical backing necessary to develop general ethical standards of medical care.

A final goal is for patients to formulate more realistic expectations about what science and medicine can accomplish. Society must face not only the economic limits that scarce health care dollars create but also the technological and human limits inherent in the empirical practice of medicine. Medicine cannot extend human lives indefinitely. Human mortality, which includes pain and suffering, disease and disability, and the certainty of death, cannot simply be conquered by "doing everything."

3. A Strategy to Achieve These Goals. An effective strategy for achieving the above goals is, first, for the public to voice concern about the overuse of medical treatments and to insist on accountability from all health professions. Second, public organizations, such at the National Institutes of Health and various Public Health Service agencies that provide important financial backing for clinical research, should be asked to assign a high priority to outcomes studies. Finally, the public must educate itself about the ethical values that underlie alternative applications of medical technologies. Rather than resorting to an anti-intellectual or anti-science mentality, or engaging in unconstructive technology-bashing, the public should seek to develop a clearer understanding of the ethical values at stake when medical techniques are put to various uses.

4. Tactics to Implement This Strategy. The media sould be reminded of its professional responsibility to assist with public education and debate. (Just as the medical profession should be taken to task whenever it puts selfish interests ahead of patients' interests, so should the media be challenged whenever it callously sensationalizes events to grab attention and sell products.) Responsible journalism can focus on dramatic cases that crystallize important issues, but should also include general discussion to identify important misconceptions and solicit input from health care leaders, lawyers, ethicists, economists, and others.

Grassroots civic and educational organizations can also mobilize the public and stimulate a clarification of values through public forums and town meetings that help citizens to wrestle with important social and ethical questions. Both of us have participated in numerous ethics conferences to provide continuing professional education for health practitioners. Both of us have also contributed to ethics conferences designed for the lay public, and sometimes broadcast over local and national radio and television stations. These conferences stimulate ethical discussions of medical ethics and are supported through grants from private and public organizations; hospitals and other health care facilities; and medical, nursing, and other health professional organizations. The so-called "Ethics in America" format broadcast in recent years over public television stations is a first-rate example of public education in spirit of "deliberative democracy," which means thoughtful and active citizenship.[19]

In summary, we call upon patients to:

1. Expect from all health care professionals a renewed commitment to patient-centered medicine. That is, expect a renewed commitment to heal the sick and help and care for suffering persons. Health professionals should be encouraged to act according to, rather than contrary to, their moral consciences. They should not prolong the dying process through efforts that merely produce physiological effects but fail to confer corresponding benefits.

2. Demand that the government, medical schools, hospitals, and other institutions direct more attention and funding to improving the hu-

mane practice of medicine. This includes both empirical research about the outcomes of treatments in different patient groups and ethics research that clarifies the values associated with alternative applications of medical technologies.

3. Accept the variety and complexity of the human condition and the inevitability of death. This requires acknowledging that there are limits to even the most advanced medical and scientific technologies. It also entails recognizing that modern medical treatments convey not only benefits but also significant psychological, spiritual, and economic burdens.

CHAPTER 9

THE WAY IT IS NOW / THE WAY IT OUGHT TO BE: FOR HEALTH PROFESSIONALS

THE WAY IT IS NOW

Dora Sauell (not her real name), a widow of some seven years, liked to spend her days bustling from one neighbor to another, keeping up with the latest gossip in the trailer park. One day she awoke with severe chest pain, called 911, and was rushed by ambulance to the emergency department of a nearby hospital, a journey that began a four-month odyssey of complications in the hospital intensive care unit until she died. On admission, a heart attack was diagnosed and treated aggressively with anticoagulants. An attempt was made at coronary angioplasty, in which a catheter is pushed into the coronary artery to open the clot, but this resulted in further damage to the heart muscle, necessitating coronary artery bypass surgery. During her recuperation, she developed massive bleeding from a stress ulcer in the stomach. This caused periodic collapses in blood pressure, further damaging her heart and leading also to kidney failure. She then developed a severe respiratory distress syndrome, rendering her unable to breathe and oxygenate her blood without the help of a mechanical ventilator. While in the intensive care unit, she required constant monitoring of blood pressure and heartbeat, correction of electrolytes and supervision of her ventilator, as well as kidney dialysis treatment two to three times a week. Because she continually spiked fevers, the doctors ordered frequent blood cultures. These required repeated punctures of veins that were harder and harder to find. Twice she suffered a cardiac arrest and on both occasions her heartbeat was restored by use of a high-voltage cardiac defibrillator. Throughout this time she had fluctuating consciousness, spending most of her time sleeping or grimacing with pain and unable to speak due to the tube in her trachea.

The nurses were in constant turmoil. They regarded their invasive intervention orders as an affront to their compassion for the woman. But whenever they tried to engage the physicians in a discussion about Mrs. Sauell's management, the doctors responded almost angrily to the challenge to their efforts. "Our job is to keep her alive," they would curtly respond.

The several specialists who visited Mrs. Sauell on a daily basis made sure that their treatments were proceeding in the best, most aggressive fashion. The kidney specialist was satisfied that the schedule of renal dialysis was replacing her lost renal function; the pulmonary specialist was satisfied that the ventilator was maintaining her oxygen level sufficiently high to be compatible with life, and that frequent suctions and occasional bronchoscopies were freeing her of obstructing secretions; the cardiologist concluded that Mrs. Sauell's heart was functioning at maximal capacity even though she was unable to leave the bed. The various specialists, therefore, saw their professional duties as being fulfilled. Mrs. Sauell, however, continued to languish in the intensive care unit bed. The problem was that even though each *individual* organ system could be maintained at a marginal level of function by constant intensive treatment, the *combination* of failing organ systems provided overwhelming empirical evidence that *the patient* had only the most negligible chance of ever being rescued from her present disaster.[1]

Finally the nurses demanded an ethics consult. After going over the patient and reviewing her medical record, the ethics consulting team reported to the committee their consensus that the patient had no reasonable chance of surviving outside the intensive care unit, that at best she would remain there indefinitely until she experienced some final terminal crisis, most likely a cardiac arrest. The consulting team recommended that life-sustaining efforts be replaced by comfort care. But then the hospital attorney and risk manager took over the committee's deliberations. They argued that if the decision to withdraw life-sustaining treatment became known to any of the patient's friends or to the public, the hospital might have to face embarrassing publicity (or, as they put it, "bad headlines"). Indeed, as long as the patient's insurance was covering the costs of treatment, the balance of benefits versus risks to the hospital clearly lay in continuing her treatment. The ethics committee voted to recommend continuing the present course of treatment.

What we have witnessed in this case is medicine run amok. Body parts are balkanized into subspecialty fiefdoms. The best interests of the hospital prevail over all else. And lost in the swirl is the patient-centered notion of medical treatment.

"The patient? That's not my department," proclaimed these masters of the kidneys, lungs, heart and other organs. Wedded to their own technologies, they confused effect with benefit.

"The patient? That's not our client," asserted the lawyer and risk manager. Seeking protective cover for the institution, they forced futile treatment to continue and became, in the words of ethicist Ruth Macklin, "enemies of patients."[2]

How did this convergence of interests — resulting in Mrs. Sauell's being subjected to months of futile treatments — come about? The physicians, of course, would cite the ideals of their profession as the force motivating their actions. "Our job is to keep her alive," they said. But John B. McKinlay sees a disturbing quality of self-interest in that idealistic proclamation: "With increasing specialization, students and practitioners may be trained to be dependent on certain practices or technologies; hence their continuing livelihood is to some extent contingent on the perpetuation of them. It is understandable, therefore, that some specialties are uncritically committed to particular interventions, and that they vigorously resist attempts to displace and sometimes even to evaluate them (surgical specialties are obvious examples)."[3]

In other words, not just a narrowly interpreted idealism but an all-too-profitable technological myopia causes specialists to be "uncritically committed to particular interventions," that is, to act like hammers and see every problem as a nail. You can easily imagine that if your specialty is running a mechanical ventilator or a kidney dialysis machine, or performing emergency coronary angioplasty, your first inclination would be to spring to action with your special skill whenever a patient's organ system starts to fail. Only the rare specialist who has the wisdom to raise her sights and view Mrs. Sauell in her entirety and join with colleagues to withhold aggressive interventions when it is evident that all of their collective efforts will not benefit the patient.

As for health professionals in general — and these include hospital attorneys and risk managers — who have been entrusted by society to base every professional action on the principle of beneficence, namely, to do only that which is in the best interests of the patient, they sometimes quite blatantly answer to other needs, as we saw in Mrs. Sauell's case. In Chapter 6, we witnessed the hypocrisy behind the refusal of the Rush Presbyterian St. Lukes Medical Center to withdraw the life-sustaining ventilator from the permanently unconscious baby, Sammy Linares. While stoutly maintaining that they could not participate in the heinous act of killing the baby, on the other hand, said the hospital authorities, they would find no difficulty in removing the ventilator if Mr. Linares, the father, obtained a court order. But if the hospital authorities were so willing to go along, why didn't *they* seek the court order? And in a similar example of sanctimony, Grace Plaza nursing home wrote in a letter to the husband of Jean Elbaum, dunning him for unwanted services, that they could not withdraw a life-sustaining feeding tube on his wife, a severely and permanently demented woman, because of "an overriding interest in continuing life support, irrespective of the patient's wishes." Yet in the very same letter the director warned: "You may be aware that New York State regulation sanctions the discharge of a patient for non-payment."[4] In other words, their "overriding" dedication to the preservation of life would not be a barrier to kicking out a woman in financial arrears and letting her die somewhere else!

Even if we accept the idealistic claims of health providers, it is becoming a matter of increasing embarrassment that physicians are failing to support all their therapeutic claims, namely, failing to justify their treatments by empirical evidence. As the physician and health policy expert David Eddy points out: "We are still relying on personal observations and uncontrolled clinical series, mixed together with heavy doses of clinical judgment, to learn the outcomes of our practices. These methods are simply not up to the task of evaluating modern medical practices." In fact, after surveying the medical literature, the Congressional Office of Technology Assessment concluded that only 10 to 20 percent of medical treatments in current use are supported by randomized trials. As a result, says Eddy, "we are uncertain about outcomes, there are wide variations in practice patterns, a large proportion of practices appear to be inappropriate, the evidence for most procedures is poor, and there are uncontrollable increases in costs."[5]

In a scathing commentary entitled "Technology Follies," the physician David Grimes takes his colleagues to task for not "requiring rigorous evidence of efficacy or validity before adoption and dissemination of new technologies." And although we have tended to concentrate on dramatic life-saving technology in our exploration of medical futility, we wish to emphasize that patient benefit should be the goal applied to all medical treatments. Reviewing a kaleidoscope of prevalent practices, including postcoital sperm survival tests of infertility, electronic fetal monitoring, episiotomy in childbirth, chemotherapeutic, immunologic, and physical methods to purge tumor cells prior to bone marrow transplantation, radial keratotomy to correct refractive errors of the eye — of all these and other new or venerable practices, Dr. Grimes asks rhetorically: "What procedures or practices are we involved in now which will rank with bloodletting as a folly of our time?" As Dr. Grimes observes, "'new' is not synonymous with 'improved.' This confusion, coupled with poor scientific standards, has squandered resources, wasted effort, and in some cases, harmed or killed our patients."[6]

Physician Stephen Schoenbaum points out that between 1980 and 1990, the procedures performed on Mrs. Sauell increased dramatically: coronary bypass surgery more than doubled and percutaneous transluminal coronary angioplasty increased more than ninefold. "One might expect that this phenomenon would be accompanied by a marked improvement in outcome for the American population." But he notes ironically that underprivileged population groups such as women and blacks, who were less likely to undergo the procedures, had at least as good a chance or better chance of survival.[7]

But desperate patients and their advocates cry: How will medicine ever discover new treatments and achieve new breakthroughs if it doesn't keep applying new interventions? Here we have to acknowledge that the medical profession, government agencies like the Food and Drug Administration, and society at large, particularly activists fighting particular diseases, often fail to draw an important distinction between treatments that empirically have already been shown to fail and therefore should be considered futile, and treatments for which there is promising but as yet insufficient supportive evidence and therefore can be regarded as *experimental*.

With respect to unproven but plausible treatments, physician-ethicist Steven Miles raises an appropriate caution:

> Our society believes that technical progress will solve tragic problems. Entrepreneurs and researchers implicitly or explicitly promise such relief. Many desperately ill persons choose to participate in creating medical progress or reaping its first, most uncertain, benefits. The recent controversy over government procedures for releasing unproven AIDS treatments for clinical use illustrates the power of these values. Permitting private purchase of nonvalidated therapies (e.g. for-profit, noninsured immunotherapy for cancer) both undercuts the definition of futility and poses a complex problem for fair access for progress itself."[8]

We would add that the confusion may stem from society's optimistic, but erroneous, belief that any new treatment that comes along is more likely to succeed than to fail. As a result, there is always enthusiasm and pressure to try a new drug or gleaming new machine just seen in a two-minute spot on the nightly news. But this assumption that something new is likely to succeed is undermined by the more sobering empirical data. To cite one important example, the Pharmaceutical Manufacturers Association reports that for every 5,000 chemically synthesized substances, only 250 reach the stage of animal testing, 5 are studied in humans, and only 1 ends up being approved by the Food and Drug Administration.[9] In short, at every step of development most new drugs are cast aside.

Physician and researcher Thomas Chalmers estimates that, with the rare exception of the discoveries of penicillin for pneumonia, vitamin B12 for pernicious anemia, insulin for diabetic acidosis, and perhaps one or two other situations in the whole history of medicine, fewer than one of a thousand new treatments introduced every year turns out to be unequivocally successful. Most are of limited or dubious or negligible benefit or indeed may be harmful.[10]

Thus, we emphasize that although patients certainly are entitled to ask their doctors for an experimental drug or procedure that is promising and undergoing clinical evaluation, they do not have a right to demand as *therapy* that for which there is no demonstrated benefit or that for which there is overwhelming empirical evidence that it will not succeed. (We distinguish between the word *treatment*, whose root meaning is to "handle" or "deal with," and *therapy*, whose root meaning is to "cure.") Once again, medications and procedures that have no demonstrated benefits are experimental until their benefits or their futility have been shown through objective, prospective, randomized clinical trials. Patients receiving unproven treatments are participating in experiments, and should be so advised by physicians when obtaining their informed consents, and they should be protected by institutional human subject review boards that monitor all research on patients.

The way it is now, this does not always happen. For, as Dr. Chalmers reports:

> Unfortunately, when a physician decides he has an exciting new therapy, he usually feels he cannot start a control trial immediately because he is not sure of the dose and the patient to select; so he does a pilot study of consecutive patients. That prevents him from ever doing a randomized controlled trial for one of three reasons: He is so impressed with the efficacy of the drug in the uncontrolled trial that he cannot do a study for ethical reasons, and he publishes his "excellent results" in a preliminary paper. He concluded that a control trial should be done but he does not do it because he is convinced that the drug works. It is often ten years before other clinical investigators, stimulated by a lack of success and less well patients report equally uncontrolled negative series or finally do a controlled trial. A second possibility is that the originator of the therapy cannot do a control trial because the treatment seems so ineffective that he cannot subject more people to it; yet it is entirely possible that it is the selection of patients who receive the treatment rather than the treatment itself that is at fault. This is especially true in the case of drastic "last resort" therapies. . . . At any rate, the therapy appears so unfavorable that a controlled trial would be unethical. The third possibility is that the therapy appears to be similar to other therapies, and the investigator has no incentive to spend his time doing a control trial to prove that a suggestive therapy is no different from the standard. . . . the only way to avoid this trap is to randomize the first patients."[11]

As we have previously noted, Mildred Solomon and her colleagues reported the astonishing fact that the majority of doctors participated in treatments that they regarded as inappropriate for terminally ill patients, which they nevertheless continued to force on their patients in spite of pangs of conscience.[12]

Because of their location in the hierarchy of power, nurses suffer particularly from this cognitive and moral dissonance. This dissonance, described as "moral distress," is the emotional suffering one undergoes when forced to act in a way that one recognizes to be wrong. The nurses caring for Mrs. Sauell were particularly vulnerable, since every day they were there at the bedside, witnesses to her misery, nausea, or incontinence; yet they were under orders to attend to her intravenous and nasogastric tubes and her mechanical ventilators, and to assist with cardiac resuscitation. Throughout their care they felt powerless to change the patient's circumstances because the physicians had ordered them to follow certain procedures and because the hospital authorities had overruled their concerns.

Nurse and researcher Judith M. Wilkinson surveyed and interviewed some two dozen hospital nurses and discovered that almost all of them had experienced this kind of moral distress at least once a week. These experiences produced anger, frustration, and guilt, and some nurses even speculated that the quality of the care they delivered was compromised. Most of the cases involved causing pain and suffering to patients and treating them in a dehumanizing way. To review their comments on the patients they cared for is in itself distressing. For example:

> The man was a century old. He would probably have gone in peace and would not have had to spend his last days this way—he has decubitus, an open sore. He has been on the ventilator, comatose, in this state forever.

> I remember crying as we cleaned her up. There was a lot of blood. They had tried to start IVs and stuff. She was oozing blood; she had started vomiting as she stopped breathing. Dark fluid . . . was coming out of her mouth. Her abdomen was distended and tight—probably full of blood. She looked bad. I just felt she should have been able to die with some kind of dignity.[13]

How do physicians get lured into prescribing treatments that offer no benefit to their patients and yet persist in pursuing these measures? Again, we go to Dr. Chalmers. He points out that as far back as 1969, physicians had information warning them that oral drugs that lowered blood glucose were more likely than either inactive placebo or insulin to cause the death of their diabetic patients. Although the prevailing idea at the time was that lowering blood glucose would save lives by reducing the rate of cardiovascular disease in patients with diabetes, a prospective clinical study showed that, quite the contrary, the drugs seemed to increase the risk of death. The results were met with great controversy and it was generally agreed that further studies were necessary. But none were undertaken. "Meanwhile," writes Dr. Chalmers, "as a result of the 'ethical practice' of medicine, gross sales of oral agents have steadily climbed. The only conclusion one can draw is that we should have had multiple studies started simultaneously when the drugs were first introduced, so we could answer the therapeutic questions before the ethical problems became insurmountable."[14]

We would add that the above is yet another example of effect-benefit confusion that is a product of physician training today. This training tends to focus on effects achieved on body parts (such as hearts, lungs and blood glucose) as distinct from benefits experienced by patients as a whole. Diabetes specialists who hypothesized that strict control of blood glucose would improve a patient's health and prolong life by preventing the complications of the disease, such as blindness, atherosclerosis, and kidney failure, apparently took for granted that it didn't matter how the blood glucose was controlled. They assumed that producing a physiological effect (lowering blood glucose) was equivalent to achieving a benefit to the patient (preventing complications and prolonging life). In fact, recent studies show that strict control of blood glucose with the use of small and frequently injected insulin does result in all these beneficial outcomes, at least to patients with the more severe (insulin-dependent) form of the disease—although perhaps not with noninsulin-dependent diabetes mellitus.[15] But the difference is that while both interventions achieve the same measurable effect, only insulin produces a benefit to the patient. Perhaps there is some unrecognized harm associated with the use of oral diabetic agents that does not occur with insulin. In any event, many diabetes specialists who were expert in the use of the oral medicines became fixated on the effects of these medicines, and resisted (sometimes with indignation) the unexpected results of the clinical trial that had showed a lack of benefit and possible harm by their favorite intervention.

THE WAY IT OUGHT TO BE

There are signs that critics within medicine are losing patience with the current state of their profession and are raising serious doubts that physicians have lived up to their ethical responsibilities. Dr. Stephen Schoenbaum, for example, states that

> it should be disturbing to us as a profession that we have so few outcomes data and use so few in our practices. . . . And although we talk about *primum non nocere* [first to do no harm] we clearly have a bias toward action. It is hard to escape the fact that we can rejoice with our patients and their families when they have good outcomes, empathize with them when they have poor outcomes, get personal gratification from the interaction and our work in both instances, and not trouble them or ourselves with hard data. In short, we learn to enjoy playing the game of medical care without hard evidence and the outcome—often unknown in statistical terms—is of secondary importance to the process.[16]

Like his colleague, Dr. McKinlay, he then issues a more devastating indictment:

> Major industries have grown up to support our practices. The industry supporting angiography—PTCA [percutaneous transluminal coronary angioplasty] and bypass surgery—range from medical equipment companies to the educational apparatus that trains all the levels of staff engaged in the decision-making and execution of these procedures to the hospitals and surgicenters whose bottom lines depend on this production. They are formidable forces with which to contend.[17]

One visible manifestation of the shift away from relying exclusively on the "bias toward action" every time a patient seeks medical help and toward examining more forthrightly whether or not the medical intervention will provide a benefit is the evolution of clinical practice guidelines. At best these guidelines are the offspring of expert panels that review the accumulated evidence associated with a particular intervention and provide a consensus statement and set of practice guidelines along with a critical appraisal of the evidence in support of the panel's recommendations.

Such guidelines are based on the notion of technology assessment, which seeks to improve the care of individual patients by gathering and analyzing information from studies carried out on large groups of patients. However, critics have faulted many of these studies for reflecting the scientific perspective of statisticians rather than the perspectives of patients. For example, a popular booklet put out by the American Heart Association reported the death rate of patients with coronary heart disease, but nowhere mentioned "the plight of the survivors — their level of disability and quality of life."

> Similarly, much technology assessment is based on physician-oriented "objective" outcomes such as physical signs and test responses, rather than patient-oriented "subjective" outcomes such as quality of life and well-being. Objective outcomes are certainly easier for investigators to measure, but subjective outcomes are arguably more relevant to individual patients."[18]

According to the American College of Physicians, "when done well — as some indisputably are — guidelines seem to represent the best possible way to collect, make sense of and then summarize for otherwise overwhelmed doctors the abundance of current research and opinion on medical procedures and outcomes."[19] The college warned, however, that nearly every group with a stake in health care is busily writing guidelines, including physician specialty societies, insurance companies, utilization reviewers, patient advocacy groups, and managed care organizations. Although the purpose of such guidelines is to provide the best and most appropriate patient care, some groups may be more interested in justifying procedures or reimbursements or cost-cutting measures or promoting business or other private interests. Therefore, it is essential that physicians demand that any expert panels provide background information to their recommendations, including whether they are based on well-controlled, randomized studies or less rigorous evidence. Equally important, physicians should require that outcome measures be couched in terms not of effects on body parts but of benefits to patients.

Dr. Bruce G. Charlton relates this new development within the profession to a growing public health orientation within medical ethics. He points out that although medical ethics has traditionally been concerned with the moral code regulating the doctor-patient relationship, public health views this relationship within the context of the community as a whole and in light of scientific measures that enhance society's health. "In public health, it is generally untrue to say that something *must* be done, because if there is no good scientific evidence of benefit, then it is better that *nothing* be done. Scientific evidence for a treatment's effectiveness should be established *before* it is introduced into the medical setting on a large scale" (italics in original).[20] We submit that the same logic applies on a small scale: When there is no scientific evidence that *something* benefits an individual patient, it is better that *nothing* be done to that patient.

It should not come as a surprise that there are those in medicine and other health care professions who are nervous about appearing in public without the clothes of the emperor. Are we really capable of looking at ourselves critically? Clearly, some of us are, for we recognize that if the public draws attention to our raiment—some sequins, some patches—before we do, embarrassment will be the least of our worries. Society rightly reacts with outrage when it senses a conspiracy to hide the truth. And although such skepticism is generally salutary, it sometimes provokes irrational reactions. In the case of medicine, these suspicions have already led to literally thousands of patients undergoing unnecessary suffering and premature death because they did not trust the medical profession or its warnings about many ruthlessly promoted quack cancer cures.

There can be little doubt that modern medicine offers powerful therapies to the sick. At the same time, much of what physicians do emerges from habit, conventional wisdom, and authority, and lacks that most valuable quality—supportive empirical evidence. Medicine today is undergoing a major change, recognizing the need "to make an orderly transition to a world based on evidence, carefully designed processes of care, and truly informed consent."[21]

There are indications also that physicians are reexamining their relationships to their patients and the goals of their practice. Sometimes these inquiries lead to startling results. Along with other researchers, we discovered that physicians do a poor job predicting what their patients would want in terms of various life-sustaining treatments.[22] The physicians are not alone; husbands and wives also are not very good at predicting what their spouses would want.[23] But even more disquieting, we discovered that physicians tend to project their own values on their patients.[24] Another group of physicians, led by Dr. John Wennberg, showed that patients facing prostatectomy who were exposed to an interactive videotape answering questions and offering patients' testimonials agreed to the surgery much less often than those patients who had only been exposed to the advice of their surgeon.[25] Thus it is clear that physicians should be sensitive not only to the values patients hold, especially where benefits are problematic, but also to the impact their own personal and professional values have on what passes for their patients' voluntary choices.

What will be the public's reaction to this demythologizing of medicine? We recognize that some segments of the public may stubbornly refuse to accept any limits placed on their demands for treatments, no matter how useless. The debate over screening mammography for breast cancer in women under the age of 50 is a good example. Although 30 years of studies have found no evidence that screening younger women saves lives—indeed the testing may cause more harm than good, since the vast majority of "positive" findings are false, leading to unnecessary anxiety while the women undergo additional procedures including breast biopsies—some advocates demand that the X-ray test be included in health care plans for younger women anyway. The declarations of Amy Langer, executive director of the National Alliance of Breast Cancer Organizations, exemplifies how easily the issue can be politically manipulated from one of medical value to one of symbolic significance. "What you have now," she argues, "is a very powerful group of women who are extremely angry and frustrated that very little is known about breast cancer." Ignoring the data in her misguided anger, she continues: "Women will not stand for the government or others to try to take away the only tool we have that is a proven intervention. Maybe it's not good enough, but it's the best we have."[26]

Thus, we see that the process of open and honest scrutiny can unleash unsophisticated outcries, which, abetted by special interests and clumsy political action, may result in more harm than good to society. But our response is first, to underscore society's right to be informed about all aspects of medical care, and, second, to be optimistic about the marketplace of ideas and hopeful that public discussion will in the long run lead an educated society to make thoughtful and worthy choices.

Already, professor of law and psychiatry Alan Meisel has seen a public consensus developing in support of medical approaches that replace aggressive, pointless treatments with an acceptance of limits and an emphasis on compassion. He points out that "the consensus about the circumstances under which it is legitimate to forgo life-sustaining treatment has become as widely accepted as it is in no small part because it has found a receptive audience among judges, legislators, and the public at large whose views lawmakers often reflect."[27]

Indeed, evidence of this can be seen in the popular press. For example, the *New York Times* recently reported approvingly:

> Already, medical researchers are trying to reduce ineffective or harmful procedures by developing guidelines on, for example, which patients will benefit from operations like coronary bypass. Insurers, through "managed care" have also tried to weed out procedures and hospital days that are not medically necessary.
>
> Pruning out inappropriate care is only sensible—but it is not rationing. Refusing to pay for something, not because it is ineffective but because its costs greatly outweigh potential benefits, would be the great departure.
>
> Not every expert agrees that rationing is needed in the foreseeable future, even if the country adopts the ceiling on spending. After studying the results of many procedures, including coronary bypass, angioplasty, hysterectomy and gall bladder operations, Dr. Robert Brook and his colleagues at the RAND Corporation concluded that one-quarter to one-third of all medical care in the country is either inappropriate or carries risks that equal potential benefits. "We have to get rid of all that before we talk about rationing," Dr. Brook said. "We have at least ten years before we have to think about rationing."[28]

Or, as Jane E. Brody, a medical writer for the *New York Times,* said, "Families as well as patients are often furious and frustrated with what they consider a lack of compassion in medicine's insistence upon prolonging a life that no longer seems worth living."[29]

It seems clear to us, therefore, that health professionals must take the lead in establishing ethical limits to their obligation to attempt treatments that empirical evidence shows are destined to be futile. Dr. David Mirvis, exhorting his medical colleagues to speak "with one voice," points out that medicine is based on a highly specialized body of knowledge that is not easily accessible to the public. "Even though the public does not fully understand what the profession does," society trusts physicians to act on behalf of the public's best interest; society looks to the institutions of medicine for the establishment of "codes of ethics, expectations of physicians' practice standards, and fundamental mechanisms for peer review, as well as basic standards of medical education." Physicians, he admonishes, "can give the patients only that which they have under their control."[30]

WHERE DO WE GO FROM HERE?

At the outset of this book we noted that although the term *futility* is actively used in medical discourse, some critics object to the concept, calling it "elusive," "unsettling," "dangerous" and devoid of a "clear sense of public values."[31] If such objections prevail, they will effectively undermine assertions made by a wide variety of authorities that physicians are not obligated to provide futile treatment.[32] Must medical futility be construed only as an ambiguous concept, cited in the abstract, or can it be defined with sufficient specificity to be useful in clinical practice?

As we have noted, much of the resistance to the notion of futility derives from the fear that it will serve as a masquerade for less defensible motivations. For example, will its acceptance revive discarded abuses of medical paternalism? Will it reverse recent advances in patient autonomy and shared decision-making? Will the power to declare treatment futile provide a convenient excuse for physicians to neglect patients they deem unworthy? Will it entice nervous health care providers to avoid patients with life-threatening contagious illness? Will futility serve as a devious rationale for reducing medical costs?

We acknowledge these potential corruptions of the concept, yet maintain that they are more likely to occur under the present state of ambiguity. Only by developing a rigorous definition of futility will clarity of thinking prevail with regard to the larger ethical problem of withholding and withdrawing medical treatment. It is particularly important, for example, to distinguish futility (implying no apparent therapeutic benefit) from rationing (acknowledging therapeutic benefit but raising questions about cost-worthiness).[33] In our experience, rationing is the notion most often confused with futility. For just as physicians find it painful to admit to a patient or family that they have run out of beneficial treatments, so too they find it difficult to upset egalitarian ideals by selectively apportioning such treatments.

Not too long ago, a period of uncertainty preceded the establishment of a uniform definition of death based on the so-called whole brain standard. After considerable debate and expert testimony within the medical, philosophical, and legal communities, most states have adopted the Uniform Brain Death Act.[34] Although it is unlikely that the definition of futility will ever be enshrined at the statutory level (nor should it, since it inherently depends on a complex variety of clinical circumstances and treatments), we suggest that therapeutic futility be defined within the context of evolving "standards of care."

Just as empirical studies are always gathering data about treatments that provide significant clinical benefits, we believe that attention should be paid also to treatments that do not provide such benefits.[35] The development of clinical predictive models in intensive care units for critically ill children and adults is an important recent medical advance that offers physicians the opportunity to forecast and distinguish with increasing accuracy survivors and nonsurvivors. Examples of such models employing various clinical and laboratory measures are the APACHE (Acute Physiology, Age, Chronic Health Evaluation) and PRISM (Pediatric Risk of Mortality).[36] These have been developed on thousands of patients, validated in many different ICUs in at least six different countries. More recently investigators have taken into account the dynamic nature of disease and added a time dimension to the scoring system to enhance the accuracy of prediction. Skeptics argue that scoring systems on seriously ill patients, though offering overall probabilities, may be limited in their power to predict futility in a particular patient. However, physicians are not limited to numerical scores in predicting futility. Many conditions cannot be overcome, and physicians could reasonably conclude at some clinical stage that there is no realistic chance the patient will benefit from aggressive treatment. Although scoring systems cannot predict a treatment outcome with absolute certainty, they provide valuable information about its likelihood. Such information would provide the empirical basis for establishing standards of care, which would refer not only to the employment of useful treatments but also to the withholding of useless ones. As standards of care serve as clinical practice guidelines to physicians and as professional standards to the court, physicians who decline to use futile treatments, even when demanded by patients and families, will be able to make these decisions with legal, as well as ethical, support.

GETTING FROM HERE TO THERE

So far we have stressed that a wide gulf exists between "the way things are" and "the way things ought to be." We now turn to the practical problem of "getting from here to there." Throughout the book, we have emphasized that changing the practice of medicine so that futile treatments are no longer applied requires the medical profession to achieve consensus about the definition of medical futility. We now wish to add the important point that, in the last analysis, society at large must understand and approve of any definition of futility and accept or reject the ethical implications proposed in this book.

The distinction we have drawn between effects and benefits requires for its application not only empirical data but also ethical assessments of when effects represent benefits or harms to patients. We can look to the empirical practice of medicine to provide information about the outcomes of various interventions in different populations. Initially, medicine and other health care professions bear the responsibility of formulating professional standards in this area.[37] These professions are accountable to the public which they serve, of course, and that must ultimately decide whether or not it agrees that particular outcomes provide an ethically acceptable likelihood or quality of benefit to persons or are futile.

In this regard it is instructive to review the debate that ensued when we called on the American Heart Association (AHA) to modify the professional standards for emergency medical service units attempting CPR and other life-prolonging treatments outside the hospital setting.[38] Under the existing AHA standards, paramedics responding to an emergency call were obligated to attempt CPR — even when it was clearly futile — unless the victim shows grossly obvious signs of death, such as decapitation, rigor mortis, or the changes of tissue decomposition and discoloration. We pointed out that in other areas of medicine, decisions are made to withhold a futile treatment without requiring that the patient be dead. Why cannot CPR decisions similarly be made in accordance with a patient-centered notion of medical futility — that is, in accordance with whether under the circumstances CPR is likely to restore the patient, at the very least, to conscious awareness? Although acknowledging that "physicians should not be obligated to provide futile therapy when asked to do so by patients or surrogates," the AHA rejected what it called a "less strict and less objective" and "looser meaning of futility." The examples it gave to counter the "less strict and less objective" application of medical futility are sadly revealing of how medicine has lost its way. CPR, states the AHA, should always be attempted in a young patient in a permanent vegetative state because even though it will not restore consciousness, it may restore circulation and therefor permit long-term survival. And, states the AHA, CPR should never be withheld unless "no survivors have been reported under given circumstances in well-designed studies" (2283).

It should be clear from these examples that terms like *strict* and *loose* are misleading. The debate over whether CPR should be undertaken to preserve a permanently unconscious body is not a matter of strict or loose criteria, but rather whether such an outcome is an appropriate goal of medicine. One can set strict criteria that focus on patient-centered benefits and exclude the goal of preserving unconscious biological existence. Similarly, the requirement that CPR be attempted unless "no survivors" have been reported in "well-designed" studies includes both an absurdity and a hidden value statement. As we have already pointed out in Chapter 1, one can never be absolutely certain under any circumstances that there will be zero survivors. Furthermore, what value assumptions are hidden in the term "well-designed" study? Does it mean one that draws conclusions after a hundred cases, a thousand cases, a million cases? At some point, common sense (we hope) will step in and say, "Enough's enough!" But when this happens, it will not be in accordance to some objective, "strict" criteria, but rather when the medical profession, supported by society, agrees that a treatment has been tried and shown not to achieve the intended benefit to the patient.

Interestingly, lawyers (more than physicians) have been in the vanguard of seeking to prevent the legal chaos of ad hoc and patchwork court decisions by establishing standards of care regarding medical futility.[39] Because courts look to statements by professional groups and institutions for definitions of standards of practice and of the legal duties to which members of the medical professions must comply, publicly stated institutional policies regarding medical futility will be important to protect and reassure physicians and those who seek to override demands for futile treatment. Otherwise, says law professor Marshal B. Kapp, "the legal system will continue to blunder along with physicians dragged in tow."[40]

In a section of a law review article, entitled "Why Hospitals Should Adopt a Policy on Futility," Professor Lance Stell states:

> Hospitals should consider adopting clear, reasonable institutional standards for withholding or withdrawing futile treatments that would serve as a local standard of care. These standards should require prompt, clear communication with the patient or his representative regarding withholding or withdrawing interventions on grounds of futility. Not to do this invites suspicion and cynicism and erodes medical integrity. In the absence of a standard, physicians who feel compelled to comply with medically unjustified demands for full measures may practice strategic concealment of their decisions or deliver half-measures in selected cases.[41]

Because all of us, both health professionals and laypeople, may at some time be patients who are subject to the definition and ethical principles that govern medical futility, we all have an essential stake in how the definition and ethical principles are developed. For these reasons, we believe health care professionals have a responsibility to contribute to the education of patients and the public at large about the meaning and ethical implications of medical futility.

In particular, society and the medical profession should not be lured into the position that "it's only a matter of money," with the implication that no standards or limits should be set, but rather that doctors should be expected to do anything, no matter how extreme and absurd, as long as someone is willing to pay for it. Apparently, as we pointed out in Chapter 5, the *New York Times* viewed the futility debate in this simplistic way when it headlined the story about a hospital's efforts to discontinue what it regarded as inappropriate life-prolonging treatment of an anencephalic infant (born with most of its brain missing): "Court Order to Treat Baby Prompts a Debate on Ethics: At What Point Does Treatment Cease to Be Worth the Expense?" Is this what the health care profession wants—to advocate, like the oldest profession, no standards other than those of the marketplace?

In proposing the quantitative component of futility, we have tried to overcome the problem of uncertainty in medicine by asking whether physicians would agree with the common sense notion that if a treatment has not benefited the patient in the last 100 cases, it would be reasonable to conclude that it is futile (upper limit of 95% confidence interval = 3%).[42] Since it comports with what has become the traditionally conservative level of medical inference of statistical significance, expressed as $p < 0.01$, it is probably not surprising that other physicians have independently arrived at a similar quantitative threshold when invoking futility on an empirical basis.[43]

We acknowledge that the actual application of the quantitative component of futility will probably vary in different communities and hospitals, since the likelihood of a patient with complex and serious illness surviving to hospital discharge following CPR will not necessarily be the same in a small rural hospital as it is in a major urban teaching center.[44] Nor will the combinations of patient characteristics associated with survival following CPR (e.g., diseases, age, gender) be the same in all hospitals.[45] However, this does not mean that the definition of futility itself varies. Nor does it mean that medical futility should be defined so loosely as to escape professional standards. We disagree, therefore, with the physician–attorney, who, because one study did not find universal predictors of cardiopulmonary resuscitation outcomes, threw up his hands and denounced the "pursuit of a clinical Grail of CPR futility."[46]

Although we do not advocate a "national futility policy" consisting of a single, universal practice guideline, we do urge that the medical profession throughout the country address the issues of medical futility's meaning and ethical implications. We propose that medical futility refers to treatments that have no reasonable chance of benefiting the patient. As we have suggested, although variables such as age, gender, and diseases may not be reliable predictors in all hospitals, they most likely will be reliable across the majority of institutions. Therefore, specific protocols for withholding and withdrawing CPR could be tailored to individual institutions, as long as professional standards of care are met.

Both quantitative and qualitative components of medical futility highlight the distinction between a treatment effect, which merely alters some part of the patient's body, and a treatment benefit, which can be appreciated by the patient and enables the patient to escape total dependence on intensive medical care. With respect to qualitative futility, a treatment that cannot provide a minimum level of benefit should be regarded as futile. Neither qualitatively futile nor quantitatively futile treatments are owed to the patient as a matter of moral duty. To the contrary, we believe that the physician has a positive duty to cease or withhold futile interventions.

We acknowledge that there is no present consensus within the medical profession about the exact dimensions of futility. We have observed, however, that this lack of consensus has not kept the term from being invoked by health providers to justify decisions concerning treatment or nontreatment. In consultations and conferences we occasionally hear futility cited when, in our view, it is not appropriate.[47] On other occasions, we fail to hear the word when the concept is in everyone's mind. Can the medical community achieve a consensus and put forward for public assessment a definition of medical futility? One answer is to point out that the courts will not await such a development, but rather they will continue to make ad hoc emotionally propelled decisions,[48] or — as in the court-ordered treatment of an anencephalic baby — decisions based on idiosyncratic interpretations of federal statutes like the Americans With Disabilities Act, the Rehabilitation Act of 1973, and the Emergency Medical Treatment and Active Labor Act (enacted to prevent hospital "dumping"),[49] causing physicians and patients to become mired in ever more intractable confusion.

Therefore, in our view, the responsibility rests with the medical profession to take the initiative by offering specific standards and guidelines in the hope of first achieving consensus within the medical community and ultimately gaining acceptance in society at large. The specific steps we propose are as follows:

1. Acknowledge that the word *futility* is widely used in medical practice, and agree to use it in a more consistent and explicit fashion than it is today.

2. Seek a specific meaning for the concept through open debate and consensus-seeking. Start with the general proposal that medical futility means treatment that fails to achieve the goals of medicine, in that it offers no benefit to the patient above a minimal quantitative or qual-

itative threshold. Then see whether the medical profession can agree as to what counts as a minimum probability or minimal quality of benefit.

3. Introduce this definition of futility into practice by encouraging publication of studies reporting not only positive therapeutic outcomes (to be adopted) but negative therapeutic outcomes (to be avoided). These empirical studies will form the basis for defining professional standards of care (also called practice guidelines) for clinical situations.

4. Seek to educate and obtain the concurrence of society at large by declaring these standards of care openly, as institutional policies for the information of the public (including legislatures and governmental agencies) and as guidelines for the courts.

CHAPTER 10

SUMMING UP:

MEDICAL

FUTILITY

In October 1992 a baby was born in a Virginia hospital with most of her brain, skull, and scalp missing — a condition called anencephaly. Because of this condition — which was recognized by ultrasound before birth — the baby, known as Baby K, will never be conscious or be able to think, see, hear, or otherwise interact with her environment. The physicians explained to Baby K's mother that the most they do for anencephalic infants is to blanket and hydrate them respectfully until they die, usually within a few days of birth. However, as soon as the newborn began to show signs of respiratory failure, the mother demanded all aggressive life-support treatments, including mechanical ventilation and cardiopulmonary resuscitation if the heart stopped. Yielding to the mother's demands, the physicians did everything they could to keep Baby K alive.

After a month of this treatment, the hospital tried to transfer Baby K to another hospital more sympathetic to the mother's wishes; however, no hospital in the area would accept the infant, and the baby was instead placed in a bed in a nearby nursing home. At the time of this writing, Baby K has survived more than a year and a half and has been readmitted to the hospital repeatedly due to breathing difficulties. Each time, on the mother's insistence, the baby has been given mechanical ventilation and other life support interventions, even though the physicians have continued to argue that such treatments are inappropriate.

After attempts to resolve the matter through the hospital ethics committee failed, the hospital requested a court declaration that the hospital not be required to provide such treatments, arguing that "because of their extremely limited life expectancy and because any treatment of their condition is futile," the standard of care is to provide comfort only.[1] However, in a series of court decisions rising to the level of the United States Court of Appeals for the Fourth Circuit, the mother's demands for continuing aggressive life-sustaining interventions were upheld. The courts cited several federal statutes, claiming that refusal to treat Baby K would violate the Americans with Disabilities Act, the Rehabilitation Act of 1973, and the Emergency Medical Treatment and Active Labor Act (which was enacted solely to prevent hospitals from "dumping" patients who were unable to pay).

This case exemplifies the crisis we face today in medical futility, and the vast gap between the goals of medicine and the strictures of the legal system. In particular, the language used by the courts in their analysis of the case illustrates the travesty that results from a failure to distinguish between an *effect* and a *benefit* of medical treatment.

For example, the court decisions (and even the amicus brief filed in support of the hospital by lawyers for the American Academy of Pediatrics and the Society of Critical Care Medicine) repeatedly refer to Baby K's "respiratory distress," a characterization which fails to recognize that the baby is incapable of experiencing any sensation, including distress. Placing the baby on a ventilator helps the lungs to pump air; however, the baby experiences no benefit from this effect of treatment. Similarly, the Americans with Disabilities Act specifies: "No individual shall be discriminated against on the basis of disability in the full and equal enjoyment of the goods, services, facilities, privileges, advantages or accommodations."[2] Clearly, in using the term *enjoyment*, Congress did not envisage application of this act to someone with no capacity to experience, much less enjoy.

Although legally applicable to only a limited jurisiction, the *Baby K* decision already has sent shudders throughout the health care system. In our own contacts with physicians and hospital administrators and lawyers, we now hear bewilderment and concerns that they, too, will be subject to such absurd demands. We hope, therefore, that before court decisions like *Baby K* lead inexorably to what we have already called Frankenstein Medical Centers, this book will provide material upon which the medical and legal professions and society at large can reflect and take preventive action.

It probably should not be surprising in this time of soaring medical costs and proliferating technology that an intense debate has arisen over the notion of medical futility. Should doctors be doing all the things they are doing—in particular, should they be attempting treatments that have little likelihood of achieving the goals of medicine? What *are* the goals of medicine? Can we agree about what constitutes failure in such medical treatment? What should the physician do and not do under such circumstances? Exploring these issues has forced us to revisit the doctor-patient relationship in a most fundamental way.[3]

IS THERE SUCH A THING AS MEDICAL FUTILITY?

If we look up the word *futility* in the *Oxford English Dictionary,* we learn that it means "leaky, vain, failing of the desired end through intrinsic defect." What then is the "failing of the desired end" in the case of medical futility? As we have pointed out in Chapter 1, some claim that the term *medical futility* has so many possible meanings that it is too elusive to define.[4]

One proposed definition of medical futility holds that futility should depend upon the likelihood of achieving *the patient's goals.* In other words, the patient is entitled to demand any outcome he or she wishes from the physician, and the physician is not entitled to judge a treatment to be futile as long as it can offer something the patient wants. This view has arisen out of the patient-autonomy movement in reaction to abuses that took place in the previous era of strong physician paternalism. And although in many respects it is an admirable view, it is clearly flawed. Physicians are *not* obligated to yield, for example, to a patient's desire for mutilating or useless surgery. As other medical ethicists state: "The shift in emphasis from physicians' paternalism to the involvement of patients in the decision-making process is not a directive for physicians to abandon their judgment. Nor should it signal the elevation of patient autonomy to an absolute."[5] If the patient's goal is to become a world champion bodybuilder with the aid of steroids, the physician is neither ethically obligated nor legally permitted to comply with the bodybuilder's request. Nor is a surgeon obligated to perform a prophylactic appendectomy to assuage a patient's fears that her recurrent abdominal pains are due to appendicitis. These are but a few of the many instances of limitations and prohibitions on the physician's duty to achieve the patient's goal. A particularly important limitation, in this era of life-as-a-TV-movie-of-the-week, is that the physician does not owe the patient a miracle.

Another proposed definition of medical futility has to do with the unacceptable likelihood of *prolonging life*. Physicians, according to this notion, cannot declare a treatment futile as long as it can prolong life, even permanently unconscious life. Those who make this claim are probably unaware that the obligation of physicians to prolong life is not supported by the classical tradition of medicine.[6] In ancient Greece and Rome, as expressed particularly through the Hippocratic writings, the physician's duties were described as assisting nature to restore health and alleviate suffering. Life and death were viewed as natural cycles; hence, any attempt to prolong life was not considered an appropriate goal of medicine. Indeed, the Hippocratic physician shunned claims of supernatural powers in order to avoid the taint of charlatanism. It was not until many centuries later, in the late Middle Ages, when religion began to play a dominant role in medical practice, and later in the seventeenth century, when scientists began to view science as a power to be exerted *against* nature, that the duty to prolong life was introduced. But it is important to keep in mind that neither theologians, nor scientists, nor for that matter anyone else prior to the modern era could ever have imagined life in the many forms it comes today, the many states between health and death that are the outcomes of modern medical treatments. Persistent vegetative state, to name just one condition describing the permanent unconsciousness of patients like Nancy Cruzan and Karen Ann Quinlan (now called permanent vegetative state), could not even be found in medical textbooks until the last decade or so. Thus, the claim that the goal of medicine is to preserve life has ambiguous meanings and dubious roots in the historical tradition of the profession.

Another proposal is that the definition of medical futility should be limited to the unacceptable likelihood of achieving any *physiological effect* on the body. According to this proposal, the physician cannot regard a treatment as futile as long as it can maintain the function of any part of the body, such as pumping blood, digesting food, forming urine, or moving air, whether the patient is conscious or in the last moments of a terminal condition. This has been presented as a "value-neutral" definition.[7] That there are those who seriously advocate this definition illustrates how much modern medicine has lost its way, how much it has become fragmented by subspecialties and technology. To choose narrow physiological criteria as the basis for the definition of medical futility is not "value-neutral," but a value *choice* that is, in our opinion, about as far from the patient-centered tradition of the medical profession as it is possible to be.

The definition of medical futility we propose is based on the fundamental notion that medical futility is the unacceptable likelihood of achieving a therapeutic *benefit* for the *patient*. Both italicized terms are important. A patient is neither a collection of organs nor merely an individual with desires. Rather, a patient (from the word meaning "to suffer") is a person who seeks the healing (meaning "to make whole") powers of the physician. The relationship between the two is central to the healing process and the goals of medicine. The physician's charge is to provide not merely an *effect* upon some part of the body but a *benefit* to the patient as a whole. Medicine today has the capacity to achieve a multitude of effects, raising and lowering blood pressure, speeding and slowing the heart, destroying cells, transplanting organs, to name but a few. But we argue that none of these effects is a benefit unless the patient has at the very least the capacity to appreciate it, a circumstance that is impossible if the patient is permanently unconscious, as in permanent vegetative state. We further argue that an effect is not a benefit if it cannot enable the patient to achieve at a minimum life goals other than complete "preoccupation" (to a use a term Plato attributed to the demigod-physician Asclepius) with the patient's illness and the treatment.

MEDICAL FUTILITY IN THEORY

We point out that the principle that physicians are not obligated to attempt futile treatment has existed not only throughout the history of medical practice but is endorsed today by a wide range of professional societies.[8] Lack of instant gratification with the short struggle to reach a definition of medical futility has caused some to plead that the term be abandoned altogether.[9] This is absurd. Medical futility is actively used in medical discourse for the very reason that it conveys a vital meaning in medical practice — some treatments fail to achieve the goals of medicine and physicians are not obligated to attempt them. It is important that we make this clear to society as well as to the profession. Medicine has great powers, but not unlimited powers. The medical profession has important obligations, but not unlimited obligations. And just as we struggled only a few decades ago to reach an acceptable definition of death, we should not be discouraged today by the difficulty in reaching a consensus on a definition of medical futility. Failing to seek a precise meaning for the term only leaves us in the present state of ambiguity, which encourages the very abuses many people fear. Physicians should not be free to invoke medical futility unless they can justify it before their peers and before society. This requires that we examine the notion, not hide from it.

THE MYTHICAL POWER OF MEDICAL FUTILITY

In ancient Greece, the *futilis* was a religious vessel that had a wide top and a narrow bottom. This peculiar shape caused the vessel to tip over easily, which made it of no practical use for anything other than ceremonial occasions. The philosopher Don Postema has pointed out that in discussing futile therapy we should be aware that the root of the term reminds us that words have a mythical power as well as a literal meaning.[10] It is possible, therefore, that sometimes unrealistic expectations and unreasonable demands for futile treatments, such as cardiopulmonary resuscitation in a cancer patient with barely hours to live, may be expressions of deep ritualistic needs. These actions in our modern time have become almost religious ceremonies. Indeed, it is not too extreme to point out that in the past, when patients sought a miracle, they went to church and prayed to God. Today they come to the hospital and demand it of the physician. Therefore, it is important to emphasize again: Physicians are not and have never been obligated to produce a miracle.

WHAT FUTILITY IS NOT

The word *futile* has to be distinguished from a variety of etymological neighbors such as *impossible* (walking to the moon is not futile, it is impossible), *implausible* (producing a full-grown infant by in vitro techniques might be possible someday, but it is implausible), and *rare* (in addition to rarity, futility carries an operational notion: success is rare, therefore attempted treatment should not be obligatory). Nor is *futile* the equivalent of *hopeless.* Hope and hopelessness are psychological reactions to objective facts. Given our individual temperaments, all of us facing the same small chance of success in a specific procedure are likely to have different reactions ranging from euphoric optimism to bleak pessimism. And although physicians regard hope as an important psychological aid in medical care, they should not invoke hope as justification for deceiving patients by misrepresenting the facts. There are better, more humane, ways to comfort patients.

QUANTITATIVE AND QUALITATIVE MEDICAL FUTILITY

In our view, medical futility has both a quantitative and qualitative component. From the writings of the Hippocratic corpus we derive its quantitative aspect: "Whenever the illness is too strong for the available remedies, the physician surely must not expect that it can be overcome by medicine. . . . To attempt futile treatment is to display an ignorance that is allied to madness."[11]

There is also a qualitative aspect to medical futility which we can trace back to the Platonic-Asclepian era. In Plato's *Republic* we find these statements: "For those whose lives are always in a state of inner sickness Asclepius did not attempt to prescribe a regime to make their life a prolonged misery. . . . A life of preoccupation with illness and neglect of work is not worth living."[12]

QUANTITATIVE FUTILITY

To pursue first the quantitative aspect of medical futility, we draw attention to the uncertainty inherent in the practice of medicine. Every medical student learns to "never say never." And philosophers of science such as Karl Popper have pointed out that, even though one sees B follow A a hundred or a thousand or even a million times, one can never be absolutely certain that the same thing will happen again. Nevertheless, as reasonable observers we inescapably begin to draw conclusions at some point in our observations. Similarly, if B has *never* followed A after many events, at some point we begin to draw conclusions about the likelihood of B following A, although again we can never be absolutely certain. This kind of common-sense empirical reasoning forms the basis for our daily living activities. More particularly, it is the basis for the clinical practice of medicine. As one classical example, the ten-day course of penicillin treatment for beta-hemolytic streptococcal pharyngitis to prevent rheumatic fever—like nearly every treatment—is based on empirical observations. But one cannot be absolutely certain the treatment will prevent rheumatic fever in every patient. Indeed, sometimes a patient develops a serious allergic reaction to the drug and almost certainly would have been better off not having taken it. But to those who demand, "Are you absolutely certain?" the answer is always, "No." But that is not the correct question. Rather, the correct question is: How many times and to what degree do we have to fail before we agree to call a treatment futile? In medicine, as in our daily affairs, we act on the basis of empirical evidence. To overcome the paralysis of uncertainty that has forced physicians to pursue the most unlikely treatments, we have proposed in this book what is nothing more than a common-sense definition of futility. Most of us probably would agree that if a treatment has not worked in the last 100 cases, almost certainly it is not going to work if it is tried again. (Statisticians can calculate that the upper limit of the 95% confidence interval is 3%.) This proposal is not an "objective" or "value-free" definition, but rather one that seeks reasonable consensus where absolute certainty is impossible and therapeutic benefit is the goal. If we can agree to call this treatment futile then the ordinary duty of the physician does not require offering it. The medical community, or society at large, may prefer longer (or shorter) odds, but in the end we all will have to accept some empirical notion of medical futility or else throw all common sense to the wind.

Is a consensus developing for medical futility? Interestingly, within the past few years, researchers have started to report empirical outcomes of life-saving treatments, ranging from the use of steroids in brain hemorrhage to cardiopulmonary resuscitation (CPR) in various clinical circumstances, including metastatic cancer and extreme prematurity.[13] In all the studies the researchers declared that when the treatment failed after a certain number of attempts, the treatment should be regarded as futile. What is striking is that the decision to call the treatment futile was made independently by these researchers (who were unaware at the time of one another's decisions) after the number of failures fell within the same range we suggested in our original proposal.[14]

QUALITATIVE FUTILITY

We submit that the goal of medicine is not merely to provide an effect upon the body, but to provide a benefit to the patient. As already noted, a patient who is permanently unconscious will never benefit from any treatment, being bereft of the capacity to appreciate any effect. Thus, any life-prolonging treatments provided for a patient in permanent vegetative state are by definition futile. We also adopt the notion attributed by Plato to Asclepius that if the treatment fails to release the patient from being "preoccupied" with the illness and incapable of achieving any other life goal, that treatment should also be regarded as futile. For example, if the best outcome physicians can achieve is to keep the patient perpetually prisoner in the intensive care unit, that outcome should not be regarded as a success, but rather as a failure to achieve the goals of medicine. Such treatment, by our definition, is futile. Note that our outcome measure is more conservative than that of researchers we cite above. They independently concluded that when life-saving treatments, ranging from the use of steroids in brain hemorrhage to cardiopulmonary resuscitation (CPR) in various clinical circumstances including metastatic cancer and extreme prematurity, failed to result in hospital discharge of the patient after a certain number of attempts, the treatment should be regarded as futile.[15] Out of caution we have proposed a more restricted definition. But this does not represent a serious disagreement. Rather it illustrates the stepwise manner in which consensus-seeking must proceed. In our view, the medical community and society at large must critically reflect upon both of these explicitly defined notions—escape from dependence on intensive care or discharge from the hospital (and others too, perhaps)—and decide which one (or perhaps more than one) specific outcome measure represents a legitimate goal of medicine.

AN ANALOGICAL ARGUMENT FOR QUANTITATIVE MEDICAL FUTILITY: THE PLACEBO

In addition to a gathering empirical consensus supporting the quantitative definition of medical futility, there is a strong analogical argument. Everyone knows about the powerful placebo effect of drugs, which in some studies has been observed to be as high as 30 percent. Let us examine the implications of this phenomenon in the context of medical futility. If there were no limits to a physician's obligations, that is, if a physician were obligated to offer any treatment that may have worked in the past or that may conceivably work, then in the absence of a proven treatment the physician would be obligated to offer a placebo. But physicians are not morally obligated to offer a placebo whenever a beneficial treatment is unavailable. There are, of course, good reasons for this. If patients knew that physicians were always going to prescribe a treatment, there would be a complete breakdown of trust. Patients could never be sure whether the physician was prescribing something specifically indicated for the condition or a placebo. Ironically, the benefit of the placebo effect of *all* drugs would probably vanish.

ETHICAL IMPLICATIONS AND PHYSICIANS' OBLIGATIONS

In addition to proposing a specific definition of futility in terms of the failure to achieve, at some minimal quantitative and qualitative threshold, the appropriate goals of medicine, we also address the question: What is the physician supposed to do when faced with a treatment that is futile?[16] We present three options to consider:

Physicians ought to be allowed to refrain from offering futile treatment, but not be obligated to do so. Under this option, the ethical implications for physicians would be analogous to therapeutic abortion. Abortion is ethically and legally permitted by society, but individual physicians are allowed to avoid offering it as a matter of personal moral choice.

Physicians ought to be encouraged to refrain from offering futile treatment, but not be obligated to do so. Under this option, the ethical implications for physicians would be analogous to maintaining patients in permanent vegetative state. Professional authorities have recommended against keeping such patients alive by medical means, but physicians are not obligated to follow such recommendations.

Physicians should be obligated to refrain from offering futile treatment. Under this option, the ethical implications for the physician would be analogous to treating patients with human immunodeficiency virus (HIV) infection. The medical profession has unequivocally imposed on its members the obligation to treat such patients. It is a declaration, not merely a recommendation, and physicians may not opt out because of personal moral objections alone.

EXCEPTIONS AND CAUTIONS

Although seeking to define and delineate the ethical implications of medical futility as precisely as possible, we recognize that medical practice calls upon us to recognize certain exceptions and cautions.

If the physician is allowed, encouraged, or required to withhold a futile treatment, does this mean the physician enjoys the privilege of withholding discussion about such treatment? Certainly physicians do not describe to patients all the many tests and treatments they have no intention of pursuing. In our view, however, there is an important distinction to be made between treatment and information. Depending on the context and patients' state of mind, patients may be entitled to information even though they are not entitled to treatments. In this regard, physicians should anticipate and recognize the concerns of patients within the particular context of medical care. A physician need not discuss the possibility of brain surgery with every patient who has a headache. On the other hand, any patient in the intensive care unit (ICU), looking around and seeing CPR being performed to the right and to the left, is quite aware that this is one of the possible treatment options. In this setting it seems quite clear to us that physicians owe it to the patient to discuss whether or not CPR will be offered. Making a decision that a treatment is medically futile does not absolve the physician of the obligation to discuss and inform the patient about what is going on in terms of the patient's condition, prognosis, and treatment options. But it would be a mistake to create an exchange which in effect has the physician stating to the patient: "CPR would be of no use in treating your disease at this point. Do you want us to do it?" As other medical ethicists have pointed out, such a communication sends a meaningless, even contradictory, message which leads to confusion and distrust in the patient.[17] Rather than assisting the patient in exercising autonomy, it actually deceives the patient and prevents the full exercise of autonomy.

What about the terminally ill patient who requests CPR to allow one last visit from a distant loved one hastening to the bedside? Even though the physician is convinced that CPR would have almost no chance of keeping the patient alive more than a day or so in the ICU, clearly the physician will want to make an exception to accommodate the short-term goal of the patient. It is important, however, to distinguish this compassionate act from an obligatory act. The physician can easily make a compassionate exception in the case of a severely burned patient or metastatic cancer patient whose request for treatment will result in a small extension of life (a clear and limited goal and small exception to the physician's duty). But in the case of permanent vegetative state, obligating the physician to accede to a request for long-term life maintenance could lead to possibly decades of futile treatment. In contrast to those who raise fears about the erosion in value of the patient, giving the physician the opportunity to view each patient as a unique person in unique circumstances enhances the value of the individual and encourages the use of appropriate medical measures rather than the useless, thoughtless pursuit of inappropriate measures.

THE IMPORTANCE OF DEFINING MEDICAL FUTILITY

In the early stages of any controversial debate, there is always a temptation to push the problem out of sight.[18] We submit there is an important heuristic value to the search for a clear definition of medical futility, whatever one emerges.[19]

First of all, the futility debate has already resulted in more clarity of thinking, particularly in distinguishing medical futility from rationing. Medical futility signifies that a treatment offers no therapeutic benefit to a patient. Rationing specifically acknowledges that a treatment *does* offer a benefit, and the issue becomes how to distribute beneficial but limited resources fairly. With rationing, the central concern is establishing criteria and priorities for qualified patients.[20] Oregon was the first state to address these kinds of rationing questions. In the Oregon plan, however, some of the treatments that are below the funding cut-off line actually represent futile treatments since they offer no therapeutic benefit. These treatments do not strictly qualify as a rationing problem since no matter how cheap or available such treatments are, there is no point to attempt them.

On the other hand, rationing decisions do have to be made about treatments such as heart transplants, renal dialysis, and other expensive and otherwise restricted treatments, because they offer clear-cut benefits to patients in need of these treatments. To clarify further the distinction: Futility decisions are made at the bedside of a specific patient, whereas rationing decisions, involving categories of patients or treatments or circumstances, inevitably should be made at a policy level in order to assure just distribution of resources.

Second, we believe that pursuing a clear-cut concept of medical futility will encourage a more aggressive search for precisely the kind of information that our medical enthusiasm has caused us to overlook. We refer to the publication of clinical trials and retrospective studies that report not only treatments that are successful, but also treatments that are *not* successful. Both kinds of data are important to the practice of medicine; both provide guidelines for physician choice.

Third, pursuing a clear concept of medical futility will oblige us to see whether or not the medical profession can achieve consensus, one which is also acceptable to society. As we have already noted, there seems to be evidence that a consensus about quantitative futility may be forming within the medical community. It was just this process of medical attention to an important ethical issue that led to today's Uniform Definition of Death Act.

BEYOND FUTILITY TO AN ETHIC OF CARE

In this book we express our concerns that much of the current futility debate has focused too narrowly on whether or not to employ particular life-saving medical treatments.[21] This has caused an important area to be neglected, not only in treatment decisions at the bedside, but in public discussions—the physician's obligation to alleviate suffering, enhance well-being, and support the dignity of the patient in the last few days of life. We urge that discussions, both in public and at the bedside, be expanded beyond "pull-the-plug" decisions to include more attention to improving doctor-nurse interactions, so that doctors who have "nothing to offer" do not walk away leaving to nurses the "nursing care"—seemingly beneath the physicians' attention. Patients and families who demand that "everything be done" may well be expressing a subtext: "Do not abandon me."

We also call upon health care professionals to seek to persuade our institutions to set aside rooms and areas enabling family members to gather around a dying patient in a setting that maximizes intimacy and dignity as opposed to the dehumanized, efficiency-oriented areas that characterize the ICU today.

We should also urge that any new national health care plan do a better job of covering comfort care in addition to supporting aggressive futile treatment.

All this will also require public education in the concepts and realities underlying the goals and practice of medicine, and the concept of medical futility.

DISTINGUISHING TREATMENT FROM EXPERIMENT

Following the arguments we have presented, it is evident that once a treatment is shown to be futile, it should no longer be offered to a patient unless done within the context of an experimental trial, which requires a reasonable hypothesis, institutional Human Subject Committee approval, and informed consent that acknowledges that the patient is participating in an experiment rather than a treatment. For example, now that CPR in metastatic cancer patients has been shown to be futile, simply flogging such patients over and over again neither benefits them nor forces medicine to look for alternatives and move forward. Either new techniques or more precise indications should be established as promising hypotheses before attempting CPR, or alternatively, more clearly defined policies emphasizing comfort care should be put in place.

PATIENTS' RIGHTS TO UNPROVEN TREATMENTS

From the arguments presented here it should also be clear that we oppose claims that patients have a right to any treatment they wish if their disease is serious and no treatment of proven benefit is available. Activists for AIDS and Alzheimer's disease have used this argument to persuade the Food and Drug Administration to change their approval policy from one of protecting the unwitting consumer to expediting drugs on a treatment basis before they have been proved to be beneficial. Although we cannot help sympathizing with the desperation motivating these patients and their advocates, we feel a sense of despair as well for the unknown multitudes of patients who will inevitably suffer as a consequence of this policy. Sanctioning dubious drugs before their therapeutic efficacy is established by careful clinical trials only *delays* the discovery of useful drugs, because it makes recruitment of patients into prospective clinical trials more difficult. Unfortunately, only a rare drug turns out to fulfill its early promise. Thus many patients, deceived into thinking that drugs provided under medical auspices must be beneficial, are actually more likely to experience harmful side effects without compensating benefits.

OBJECTIONS TO MEDICAL FUTILITY

We shall now report and comment on a few objections that have been raised either to the very notion of medical futility, or to our specific definition of futility, or to our view of its ethical implications.

The philosopher, Daniel Callahan says that "the debate on the meaning of futility is still in its infancy. We have no clear sense of public values on these matters, no good figures on costs, no clear criteria for cost benefit calculations, and no political process to allow physicians and lay people to gather together to develop appropriate standards."[22] Callahan blurs futility with cost-containment and rationing when he mixes in cost and cost-benefit calculations. But he is right that at the present time, we have no political process to allow physicians and laypeople to explore and debate this issue. Indeed, in a letter to us, Callahan described his statement as intending to emphasize "the need to see this as a political issue as much as an ethical and medical one." In the letter, Callahan goes on to say: "In short, I am *totally* on your side about the need for futility standards, believe that appropriate procedures could be easily set up to determine them, believe also that a consensus could be reached, and that the consensus could (and should) command the support of physicians and lay people" (emphasis in the original).[23]

The law professor and medical ethicist Alexander Capron says that the definition of medical futility presented here "rests on a view that merely preserving permanent unconsciousness or failing to end total dependence on intensive medical care are ends inherently outside legitimate medical practice. Yet as the Wanglie case makes apparent, people value other outcomes."[24] Helga Wanglie was a patient in permanent vegetative state (see Chapter 4). Her husband insisted that she be maintained, treated, and resuscitated if necessary over the objections of her medical providers who sought to discontinue what they regarded as inappropriate medical treatment. Apparently, Capron is pressing the notion that physicians must give to patients whatever they seek, granting to people who "value other outcomes" a right to override "legitimate medical practice." We argue that this would make physicians unique among the professions in the extent to which they are obligated to yield to the persons they serve. Let us look, for a moment, at Capron's profession, the law. A murderer deserves a full and vigorous defense by an attorney. Does that mean that after conviction and life sentence, the permanently incarcerated prisoner can demand that the attorney phone the governor every day in search of clemency—an event that is much more likely to occur than the restoration of consciousness in a patient in permanent vegetative state? Surely at some point the lawyer would declare a limit to professional obligations to the client. Similarly, we do not think that physicians, after they have carried out their best efforts yet failed to restore a patient's consciousness, should be held obligated to continue to treat on a daily basis that patient condemned to a life sentence of unconsciousness.

The intensive care specialist physician Robert Truog and his colleagues have called for an abolition of the "language of futility": "The notion of futility generally fails to provide an ethically coherent ground for limiting life-sustaining treatment, except in circumstances in which narrowly defined physiologic futility [which they call "value-free"] can be plausibly invoked."[25]

We have already pointed out the absurdity of describing any definition of futility, but most assuredly "physiologic futility," as "value-free." Curiously, these authors try to dismiss the notion of quantitative futility when they state that, "even in theory, statistical inferences about what might happen to groups of patients do not permit accurate predictions of what will happen to the next such patient."[26] But as we have already pointed out, statistical inferences, that is, uncertainty, underlie all empirical decision-making. Their objections would lead to the dismissal of the basis of all medical practice, not to mention the empiric basis on which we conduct our daily affairs.

THE NEXT STEPS

First of all, we should acknowledge that medical futility is not something that can be dismissed from the discourse of health care providers. It has meaning and is widely used. Our challenge is to use the term in a more consistent and explicit fashion than it is today. We have observed that many times in the medical setting the term is abused because there is no standard for applying it. Physicians have invoked the term for a variety of unjustifiable reasons, ranging from a fear of being exposed to HIV infection to an objection to providing costly therapies.[27]

Second, we should explore the implications of an explicit definition of futility in medical practice by encouraging publication of studies reporting not only positive therapeutic outcomes (to be adopted) but also negative therapeutic outcomes (to be avoided). Medical practice requires a knowledge of not only what works but also what doesn't work.

Third, we hope that books and articles like this will provide the stimulus for the medical profession and the community at large to engage in education and open debate. From this process may emerge a consensus similar to that achieved with respect to the Uniform Definition of Death Act. We propose that we start with a *patient-centered* notion of medical futility, meaning a treatment that offers no benefit to the patient above a minimum quantitative and qualitative threshold. Then comes the fine tuning — can the medical profession and ultimately society agree as to where to draw the line at a minimum probability or minimum quality of benefit? In other words, how many times and to what degree should we have to fail before we agree to call a treatment futile?

Fourth, we propose that empirical studies as well as consensus agreements then form the basis for establishing standards of care. These standards of care should be declared openly as institutional policies by medical centers and organizations of medicine for the information of the public and as guidelines to the court. This last point is extremely important. Right now, as we have warned, physicians practice and patients receive treatment in an environment where ad hoc and often capricious decisions are rendered according to no agreed standards. Patients and patients' families have been forced to pay for inhumane, unwanted care either because of an individual physician's misguided notions of medical duty or as a result of hasty, ill-conceived court decisions. Physicians have practiced "defensive medicine," fearing that anything less than mindless continuation of aggressive treatments would make them legally vulnerable. As a consequence, they have given the courts little guidance but to "do everything possible."

The debate on medical futility can lead to a fresh revisiting of the doctor-patient relationship and with it a restoration of common sense and reality to society's perception of the powers of medicine. We hope also that it will bring into better synchrony the desires of patients and the hopes of families with the appropriate ends of medicine.

CHAPTER I: ARE DOCTORS SUPPOSED TO BE DOING THIS?

1. Multi-Society Task Force on Persistent Vegetative State, "Medical Aspects of the Persistent Vegetative State," *NEJM* 330 (1994): 1499–1508, 1572–79. This document provides a comprehensive update and recommends distinctions in terminology. The task force defines the vegetative state as "a condition of complete unawareness of the self and the environment accompanied by sleep-wake cycles with either complete or partial preservation of hypothalamic and brain stem autonomic functions." The task force distinguishes between the diagnostic entity *persistent* vegetative state, which refers to the clinical condition if it persists for at least one month, and *permanent* vegetative state which carries prognostic implications of irreversibility. Permanent vegetative state is "an irreversible state, a definition, as with all clinical diagnoses in medicine, based on probabilities, not absolutes." The task force states that a persistent-vegetative-state patient "becomes permanently vegetative when the diagnosis of irreversibility can be established with a high degree of clinical certainty, i.e., when the chance of regaining consciousness is exceedingly rare." Throughout this book we will refer to the vegetative state in terms that are consistent with the task force's recommendations.

2. *Cruzan v. Director, Missouri Department of Health,* 110 S. Ct. 2841 (1990).

3. *Cruzan v. Harmon,* 760 S.W. 2d 408 (Mo. 1988), cert. granted sub nom. *Cruzan v. Director, Missouri Dept. of Health* et al. 106 L. Ed 2d 587, 109 S. Ct. 3240 (1989).

4. *In re Torres,* 357 N.W. 2d, 341.

5. J. Cruzan, personal communication.

6. G. J. Annas, "The Long Dying of Nancy Cruzan," *Law, Medicine, and Health Care* 19 (1991): 52–59.

7. See note 1 above.

8. We acknowledge that some observers attribute the change in attitude to a technological advance, namely the introduction of percutaneous endoscopic gastrostomy (placing the feeding tube through the abdominal wall directly into the stomach). This procedure can be carried out easily under local anesthesia and is more comfortable for the patient. In our view, however, this causal argument is not persuasive, since patients in permanent vegetative state are incapable of feeling pain or removing any tube and could have been readily kept alive by being fed through a nasogastric tube.

We believe it is more likely that the attitude and the technology evolved concurrently and interdependently.

9. For a while, terms such as *irreversible coma, cerebral death, irreversible cessation of cerebral function,* and *coma depasse* were used to describe the ambiguous state between permanent unconsciousness and death that presented in a patient whose electroencephalogram (EEG) showed no evidence of cerebral activity. Interestingly, despite the absence of universal agreement on criteria for withdrawing mechanical aids to respiration and circulation, the *Journal of the American Medical Association* was able to report in 1969 that "no one has encountered any medicolegal difficulties. Very few have sought legal opinions." D. Silverman, M. G. Saunders, R. S. Schwab, and R. L. Masland, "Cerebral Death and the Electroencephalogram: Report of the Ad Hoc Committee of the American Electroencephalographic Society on EEG Criteria for Determination of Cerebral Death," *JAMA* 209 (1969): 1505–10.

10. N. Dubler and D. Nimmons, *Ethics on Call* (New York: Harmony Books, 1992).

11. Hippocrates, "The Art," in *Ethics in Medicine: Historical Perspectives and Contemporary Concerns,* ed. S. J. Reiser, A. J. Dyck, and W. J. Curran (Cambridge: MIT Press, 1977).

12. D. W. Amundsen, "The Physician's Obligation to Prolong Life: A Medical Duty without Classical Roots," *Hastings Center Report* 8 (1978): 23–30.

13. See note 11 above.

14. A. A. Lyons and R. J. Petrucelli, *Medicine: An Illustrative History* (New York: Abradele Press, Harry Abrams, 1987), 291.

15. N. S. Jecker, "Knowing When to Stop: The Limits of Medicine," *Hastings Center Report* 21 (1991): 5–8, at 6.

16. D. W. Amundsen, personal communication.

17. J. D. Lantos, P. A. Singer, R. M. Walker, et al., "The Illusion of Futility in Clinical Practice," *American Journal of Medicine* 87 (1989): 81–84.

18. R. D. Truogh, A. S. Brett, and J. Frader, "The Problem with Futility," *NEJM* 326 (1992): 1560–64.

19. M. Angell, "The Case of Helga Wanglie," *NEJM* 325 (1991): 511–12.

20. H. Brody, "The Power to Determine Futility," in *The Healer's Power* (New Haven: Yale University Press, 1992), 179.

21. Ibid.

22. D. Hume, *A Treatise of Human Nature,* ed. L. A. Selby-Bigge (New York: Oxford University Press, 1978), 73.

23. K. R. Popper, *The Logic of Scientific Discovery* (New York: Basic Books, 1961). With respect to the "idol of certainty," Popper states: "The old scientific ideal of *episteme* — of absolutely certain, demonstrable knowledge — has proved to be an idol. The demand for scientific objectivity makes it inev-

itable that every scientific statement must remain *tentative for ever.* It may indeed be corroborated, but every corroboration is relative to other statements which, again, are tentative. Only in our subjective experiences of conviction, in our subjective faith, can we be 'absolutely certain.'"

24. J. D. Lantos, S. H. Miles, M. D. Silverstein, and C. B. Stocking, "Survival after Cardiopulmonary Resuscitation in Babies of Very Low Birthweight: Is CPR Futile?" *NEJM* 318 (1988): 91–95; A. L. Kellerman, D. R. Staves, and B. B. Hackman, "In-Hospital Resuscitation Following Unsuccessful Prehospital Advanced Cardiac Life-Support: 'Heroic Efforts' or an Exercise in Futility?" *Annals of Emergency Medicine* 17 (1988): 589–94; M. J. Bonnin and R. A. Swor, "Outcomes in Unsuccessful Field Resuscitation Attempts," *Annals of Emergency Medicine* 18 (1989): 507–12; D. J. Murphy, A. M. Murray, B. E. Robinson, and E. W. Campion, "Outcomes of Cardiopulmonary Resuscitation in the Elderly," *Annals of Internal Medicine* 111 (1989): 199–205; K. Faber-Langendoen, "Resuscitation of Patients with Metastatic Cancer: Is Transient Benefit Still Futile?" *Archives of Internal Medicine* 151 (1991): 235–39; W. A. Gray, R. J. Capone, and A. S. Most, "Unsuccessful Emergency Medical Resuscitation: Are Continued Efforts in the Emergency Department Justified?" *NEJM* 325 (1991): 1393–98.

25. Plato, *Republic,* bk. 3, trans. E. Hamilton and H. Cairns (Princeton: Princeton University Press, 1980).

26. D. Postema, personal communication.

27. Ibid.

28. A. R. Jonsen, personal communication.

29. D. Rothman, "Strong Medicine: The Ethical Rationing of Health Care," *New York Review of Books* 39 (1992): 32–38, at 33.

30. R. Dworkin, *Life's Dominion* (New York: Random House, Vintage Books, 1994), 28.

CHAPTER 2: WHY IT IS HARD TO SAY NO

1. M. Nussbaum, "Transcending Humanity," in *Love's Knowledge* (New York: Oxford University Press, 1990), 365.

2. D. Callahan, *The Troubled Dream of Life* (New York: Simon and Schuster, 1993), 61.

3. H. Brody, "Assisted Death: A Compassionate Response to a Medical Failure," *NEJM* 327 (1992): 1385.

4. K. Lebacz, "Humility in Health Care," *Journal of Medicine and Philosophy* 17 (1992): 291.

5. L. J. Schneiderman, "Exile and PVS," *Hastings Center Report* 20, no. 3 (1990): 5.

6. J. M. Kriett and M. P. Kaye, "The Registry of the International Soci-

ety for Heart Transplantation: Seventh Official Report, 1990," *Journal of Heart Transplantation* 9, no. 4 (1990): 323–30; ibid., "Eighth Official Report, 1991," Journal of Heart Transplantation 10, no. 4 (1991): 491–98; P. M. Park, "The Transplant Odyssey," *Second Opinion* 12 (1989): 27–32; K. Rolles, "Summary of Clinical Data: Liver Transplantation," in *Organ Transplantation: Current Clinical and Immunological Concepts*, ed. L. Brent and R. A. Sells (London: Balliere Tindall, 1989), 201–5.

7. W. Cather, *Death Comes to the Archbishop* (New York: Alfred A. Knopf, 1951), 170.

8. J. Itami, "A Director Boasts of His Scars, and Says He Is Right about Japan's Mob," *New York Times,* Aug. 30, 1992, E7.

9. *The Compact Edition of the Oxford English Dictionary* (New York: Oxford University Press, 1971), 714.

10. F. W. Hafferty, *Into the Valley: Death and the Socialization of Medical Students* (New Haven: Yale University Press, 1991), 38.

11. N. S. Jecker and L. J. Schneiderman, "Is Dying Young Worse Than Dying Old?" *Gerontologist* 3, no. 1 (1994): 66–72.

12. G. J. Annas, "Faith (Healing), Hope, and Charity at the FDA: The Politics of AIDS Drug Trials," in *AIDS and the Health Care System,* ed. L. O. Gostin (New Haven: Yale University Press, 1990), 183–94, at 194.

13. See note 1 above.

CHAPTER 3: WHY WE MUST SAY NO

1. M. Z. Solomon, L. O'Donnell, B. Jennings, V. Guilfoy, et al., "Decisions Near the End of Life: Professional Views on Life-Sustaining Treatments," *American Journal of Public Health* 83, no. 1 (1993): 14–23, at 19.

2. *Barber v. Los Angeles County Superior Court,* 195 Cal. Rptr. 484, 147 Cal. App. 3d 1006 (1983).

3. Solomon et al., "Decisions Near the End of Life," at 19.

4. D. Humphry, *Final Exit* (Eugene, Ore.: Hemlock Society, 1991).

5. G. J. Annas, "Adding Injustice to Injury: Compulsory Payment for Unwanted Treatments," *NEJM* 327 (1992): 1885–87.

6. G. D. Lundberg, "American Health Care System Management Objectives: The Aura of Inevitability Becomes Incarnate," *JAMA* 269 (1993): 2554–55.

7. *New York Times,* Aug. 17, 1993, A8.

8. D. Callahan, *Setting Limits: Medical Goals in an Aging Society* (New York: Simon and Schuster, Touchstone Edition, 1988), 171.

9. J. K. Iglehart, "The American Health Care System: The End Stage Renal Disease Program," *NEJM* 328 (1993): 366–71, at 371.

10. R. M. Dworkin, "The Price of Life," *Los Angeles Times,* Aug. 29, 1993, M1.

11. Alison Taunton-Rigby, Genzyme's senior vice-president of therapeutics, quoted in "New Drug Standard: Economic Value," *New York Times,* Jan. 18, 1993, C3.

12. K. Faber-Langendoen, A. L. Caplan, and P. B. McGlave, "Survival of Adult Bone-Marrow Transplant Patients Receiving Mechanical Ventilation: A Case for Restricted Use," *Bone Marrow Transplantation* 12 (1993): 501–7.

13. S. C. Schoenbaum, "Toward Fewer Procedures and Better Outcomes," *JAMA* 269 (1993): 794–96.

14. T. S. Kuhn, *The Structure of Scientific Revolutions* (Chicago: University of Chicago Press, 1970).

15. D. Oken, "What to Tell Cancer Patients: A Study of Medical Attitudes," *JAMA* 175 (1961): 1120–28.

16. D. H. Novack, R. Plumer, R. L. Smith, H. Ochitill, et al., "Changes in Physicians' Attitudes toward Telling the Cancer Patient," *JAMA* 241 (1979): 897–900.

17. The revered physician's advice came from an honored tradition. Oliver Wendell Holmes wrote, "Your patient has no more right to all the truth you know than he has to all the medicine in your saddlebags. . . . He should get only just so much as is good for him. . . . It is a terrible thing to take away hope, every earthly hope, from a fellow creature." In "The Young Practitioner," *Medical Essays,* vol. 9, *Writings of Oliver Wendell Holmes* (Boston: 1891), 388.

18. N. S. Jecker, "The Role of Intimate Others in Medical Decision-Making," *Gerontologist* 30 (1990): 65–71; H. H. Hiatt, "Protecting the Medical Commons: Who Is Responsible?" *NEJM* 293 (1975): 235–41; G. Hardin, "The Tragedy of the Commons," *Science* 162 (1968): 1243–48; J. Hardwig, "What about the Family?" *Hastings Center Report* March/April (1990): 5–10.

19. N. S. Jecker, "Being a Burden on Others," *Journal of Clinical Ethics* 4 (1993): 16–20.

CHAPTER 4: FAMILIES WHO WANT EVERYTHING DONE

1. N. S. Weiss, J. M. Liff, C. L. Ure, J. H. Ballard, G. H. Abbott, and J. R. Daling, "Mortality in Women Following Hip Fracture," *Journal of Chronic Disease* 36 (1983): 879–82; C. W. Miller, "Survival and Ambulation Following Hip Fracture," *Journal of Bone and Joint Surgery* 60-A (1978): 930–34; B. L. White, W. D. Fisher, and C. A. Laurin, "Rate of Mortality for Elderly Patients after Fracture of the Hip in the 1980s," *Journal of Bone and*

Joint Surgery 69-A (1987): 1335–39; S. R. Cummings, D. M. Black, and S. M. Rubin, "Lifetime Risks of Hip, Colles', or Vertebral Fracture and Coronary Heart Disease among White Postmenopausal Women," *Archives of Internal Medicine* 149 (1989): 2445–48.

2. S. H. Miles, "Informed Demand for 'Nonbeneficial' Medical Treatment," *NEJM* 325 (1991): 512–15.

3. Ibid.

4. Ibid.

5. R. E. Cranford, "Helga Wanglie's Ventilator," *Hastings Center Report* July/August (1991): 23–24.

6. E. H. Cassem, personal communication. See also T. A. Brennan, "Ethics Committees and Decisions to Limit Care," *JAMA* 260 (1988): 803–7.

7. N. Daniels, *Am I My Parents' Keeper?* (New York: Oxford University Press, 1988), viii.

8. J. J. Paris and F. E. Reardon, "Physician Refusal of Requests for Futile or Ineffective Interventions," *Cambridge Quarterly of Health Care Ethics* 2 (1992): 127–34, at 127.

9. M. Angell, "The Case of Helga Wanglie: A New Kind of 'Right to Die' Case," *NEJM* 325 (1991): 511–12; A. M. Capron, "*In re:* Helga Wanglie," *Hastings Center Report* 21 (1991): 26–28; F. Ackerman, "The Significance of a Wish," *Hastings Center Report* 20 (1991): 27–29; S. M. Wolf, "Conflict between Doctor and Patient," *Law, Medicine, and Health Care* 16, no. 3–4 (1988): 197–203; T. A. Brennan, "Silent Decisions: Limits of Consent and the Terminally Ill Patient," *Law, Medicine, and Health Care* 16, no. 3–4 (1988): 204–9.

10. Paris and Reardon, "Physican Refusal of Requests," 128.

11. A. S. Brett and L. B. McCullough, "When Patients Request Specific Interventions," *NEJM* 315 (1986): 1347–51, at 1349.

12. E. Pellegrino, "Ethics in AIDS Treatment Decisions," *Origins* 19 (1990): 539–44; D. W. Brock and S. A. Wartman, "When Competent Patients Make Irrational Choices," *NEJM* 322 (1990): 1595–99.

13. J. R. Zuckerman, letter to editor, *New York Times,* Aug. 22, 1992, Y14.

14. R. M. Veatch and C. M. Spicer, "Medically Futile Care: The Role of the Physician in Setting Limits," *American Journal of Law and Medicine* 18, no. 1–2 (1992): 15–36, at 17.

15. L. J. Schneiderman, K. Faber-Langendoen, and N. S. Jecker, "Beyond Futility to an Ethic of Care," *American Journal of Medicine* 96 (1994): 110–14.

16. U.S. Department of Health and Human Services, Agency for Health Care Policy and Research, Clinical Practice Guideline, *Acute Pain Management: Operative or Medical Procedures and Trauma* (Rockville, Md.:

Agency for Health Care Policy and Research, 1992); S. Hauerwas, "Care," in *Encyclopedia of Bioethics,* vol. 1, ed. Warren T. Reich (New York: Free Press, 1978), 145–50; A. R. Nelson, "Humanism and the Art of Medicine: Our Commitment to Care," *JAMA* 262 (1989): 1228–30.

17. N. S. Jecker and J. D. Self, "Separating Care and Cure: An Analysis of Historical and Contemporary Images of Nursing and Medicine," *Journal of Medicine and Philosophy* 16 (1991): 285–306; S. A. Gadow, "Nurse and Patient: The Caring Relationship," in *Caring, Curing, Coping: Nurse, Physician, Patient Relationships,* ed. Ann Bishop and John Scudder (Birmingham: University of Alabama Press, 1985), 31–43.

18. N. S. Jecker, "Justice and the Private Sphere," *Public Affairs Quarterly* 8 (1994): 255–66. L. Blum, "Care," in *The Encyclopedia of Ethics,* vol. 1, ed. L. C. Becker and C. B. Becker (New York: Garland Publishing, 1992), 125.

19. N. Coyle, "Continuity of Care for the Cancer Patient with Chronic Pain," *Cancer* 63 (1989): 2289–93; T. D. Walsh, "Continuing Care in a Medical Center: The Cleveland Clinic Foundation Palliative Care Service," *Journal of Pain and Symptom Management* 5, no. 5 (1990): 273–78.

20. L. A. Printz, "Terminal Dehydration: A Compassionate Treatment," *Archives of Internal Medicine* 152 (1992): 697–700; P. Schmitz and M. O'Brien, "Observations on Nutrition and Hydration in Dying Cancer Patients," in *By No Extraordinary Means,* ed. J. Lynn (Bloomington: Indiana University Press, 1986), 29–38.

21. R. J. Sullivan, "Accepting Death without Artificial Nutrition or Hydration," *Journal of General Internal Medicine* 8 (1993): 220–24.

22. T. E. Quill, "Doctor, I Want to Die; Will You Help Me?" *JAMA* 270 (1993): 870–73, at 871.

23. K. Faber-Langendoen, "Medical Futility: Values, Goals, and Certainty," *Journal of Laboratory and Clinical Medicine* 120 (1992): 831–35.

CHAPTER 5: FUTILITY AND RATIONING

1. E. J. Ziegler, C. J. Fisher, Jr., C. L. Sprung, et al., "Treatment of Gram-Negative Bacteremia and Septic Shock with HA-1A Human Monoclonal Antibody against Endotoxin: A Randomized, Double-Blind, Placebo-Controlled Trial," *NEJM* 324 (1991): 429–36; H. S. Warren, R. L. Danner, and R. S. Munford, "Anti-Endotoxin Monoclonal Antibodies," *NEJM* 326 (1992): 1153–57; R. P. Wenzel, "Anti-Endotoxin Monoclonal Antibodies: A Second Look," *NEJM* 326 (1992): 1151–53.

2. K. A. Schulman, H. A. Glick, H. Rubin, and J. U. Eisenberg,

"Cost-Effectiveness of HA-1 A Monoclonal Antibody for Gram-Negative Sepsis," *JAMA* 266 (1991): 3466–71.

3. R. Pear, "Health-Care Costs Up Sharply Again, Posing New Threat," *New York Times,* Jan. 5, 1993, A1.

4. E. Ginzberg, "A Hard Look At Cost Containment," *NEJM* 316 (1987): 1151–54.

5. M. McGregor, "Technology and the Allocation of Resources," *NEJM* 320 (1989): 118–20.

6. L. J. Blackhall, "Must We Always Use CPR?" *NEJM* 17 (1987): 1281–84.

7. T. Tomlinson and H. Brody, "Ethics and Communication in Do-Not-Resuscitate Orders," *NEJM* 318 1988: 43–46.

8. J. Risen, "Expert Panel Brews Bitter Tonic for U.S. Fiscal Malaise," *Los Angeles Times,* Aug. 30, 1992, A10.

9. D. Callahan, *Setting Limits: Medical Goals in an Aging Society* (New York: Simon and Schuster, 1987).

10. We draw upon a number of studies in making these claims, including, but not limited to: D. J. Murphy, A. M. Murray, B. E. Robinson, et al., "Outcomes of Cardiopulmonary Resuscitation in the Elderly," *Annals of Internal Medicine* 111 (1989): 199–205; B. J. Gersh, R. A. Kronmal, R. L. Frye, et al., "Coronary Arteriography and Coronary Artery Bypass Surgery: Morbidity and Mortality in Patients Ages 65 Years and Older," *Circulation* 67 (1983): 483–91; T. Randall, "Successful Liver Transplantation in Older Patients Raises New Hopes, Challenges, Ethics Questions," *JAMA* 264 (1990): 428–30; J. D. Pirsch, R. J. Stratta, M. J. Armbrust, et al., "Cadaveric Renal Transplantation with Cyclosporine in Patients More Than 60 Years of Age," *Transplantation* 47 (1989): 259–61; M. P. Hosking, M. A. Warner, C. M. Lobdell, et al., "Outcomes of Surgery in Patients 90 Years of Age or Older," *JAMA* 261 (1989): 1909–15; C. B. Begg, J. L. Cohen, J. Ellerton, "Are the Elderly Predisposed to Toxicity from Cancer Chemotherapy?" *Cancer Clinical Trials* 3 (1980): 369–74; L. Westlie, A. Umen, S. Nestrud, et al., "Mortality, Morbidity, and Life Satisfaction in the Very Old Dialysis Patient," *Transactions of the American Society of Artificial Internal Organs* 30 (1984): 21–30.

11. N. Daniels, *Am I My Parents' Keeper?* (New York: Oxford University Press, 1988).

12. R. M. Veatch, *A Theory of Medical Ethics* (New York: Basic Books, 1981).

13. A. S. Brett and L. B. McCullough, "When Patients Request Specific Interventions," *NEJM* 315 (1986): 1347–51.

14. J. Hammond and C. G. Ward, "Decisions Not to Treat: 'Do-Not-Resuscitate' Order for the Burn Patient in the Acute Setting," *Critical Care*

Medicine 17 (1989): 136–38; J. D. Lantos, S. H. Miles, M. D. Silverstein, and C. B. Stocking, "Survival after Cardiopulmonary Resuscitation in Babies of Very Low Birthweight: Is CPR Futile Therapy?" *NEJM* 318 (1988): 91–95; G. E. Taffet, T. A. Teasdale, and R. J. Luchi, "In-Hospital Cardiopulmonary Resuscitation," *JAMA* 260 (1988): 2069–72; D. J. Murphy, "Do-Not-Resuscitate Orders: Time for Reappraisal in Long-Term Care Institutions," *JAMA* 260 (1988): 2098–2101; L. J. Schneiderman and R. G. Spragg, "Ethical Decisions in Discontinuing Mechanical Ventilation," *NEJM* 318 (1988): 984–88; J. J. Paris, R. K. Crone, and F. Reardon, "Physicians' Refusal of Requested Treatment: The Case of Baby L," *NEJM* 322 (1990): 1012–15; D. V. Schapira, J. Studnicki, D. D. Bradham, et al., "Intensive Care, Survival, and Expense of Treating Critically Ill Cancer Patients," *JAMA* 269 (1993): 783–86.

15. President's Commission for the Study of Ethical Problems in Medicine and Biomedical and Behavioral Research, *Securing Access to Health Care,* vol. 1 (Washington, D.C.: Government Printing Office, 1983), 46–47.

16. White House Domestic Policy Committee, *The President's Health Security Plan* (New York: Time Books, 1993).

17. R. M. Dworkin, "Will Clinton's Health Care Plan Be Fair?" *New York Review of Books,* Jan. 13, 1994, 21.

18. C. Gilligan and S. Pollak, "The Vulnerable and the Invulnerable Physician," in *Mapping the Moral Domain,* ed. C. Gilligan, J. V. Ward, and J. M. Taylor (Cambridge: Harvard University Press, 1988), 245–62.

19. Ibid.

20. N. Daniels, "Why Saying No to Patients in the United States Is So Hard," *NEJM* 314 (1986): 1380–83.

CHAPTER 6: MEDICAL FUTILITY IN A LITIGIOUS SOCIETY

1. R. F. Weir and L. Gostin, "Decisions to Abate Life-Sustaining Treatment for Nonautonomous Patients," *JAMA* 264 (1990): 1846–53.

2. L. J. Nelson and R. E. Cranford, "Legal Advice, Moral Paralysis, and the Death of Samuel Linares," *Law, Medicine, and Health Care* 17, no. 4 (1989): 316–24.

3. "America's Parasite Economy," *Economist,* Oct. 10, 1992, 21.

4. B. McCormick, "Study: Defensive Medicine Costs Nearly $10,000,000,000," *American Medical News,* Feb. 15, 1993, 4.

5. R. S. Bell and J. W. Loop, "The Utility and Futility of Radiographic Skull Examination for Trauma," *NEJM* 284 (1971): 236–39.

6. Committee to Study Medical Professional Liability and the Delivery of Obstetrical Care, Division of Health Promotion and Disease Preven-

tion, Institute of Medicine, *Medical Professional Liability and the Delivery of Obstetrical Care,* 1 (1989): 81.

7. P. W. Huber, *Galileo's Revenge: Junk Science in the Courtroom* (New York: Basic Books, 1993), 87.

8. J. H. Ferguson, M. Dubinsky, and P. J. Kirsch, "Court-Ordered Reimbursement for Unproven Medical Technology," *JAMA* 269 (1993): 2116–21.

9. *Daubert v. Merrell Dow Pharmaceuticals,* 113 S. Ct. 2786 (1993); G. J. Annas, "Scientific Evidence in the Courtroom: The Death of the Frye Rule," *NEJM* 330 (1994): 1018–21; J. E. Bertin and M. S. Henifin, "Science, Law, and the Search for Truth in the Courtroom: Lesson from *Daubert v. Merrell Dow*," *Journal of Law, Medicine, and Ethics* 22, no. 1 (1994): 6–20.

10. A. R. Localio, A. G. Lothers, J. M. Bengtson, L. E. Hebert, et al., "Relationship between Malpractice Claims and Caesarean Delivery," *JAMA* 269 (1993): 366–73.

11. Huber, *Galileo's Revenge,* 179.

12. G. Kolata, "Patients' Lawyers Lead Insurers to Pay for Unproven Treatments," *New York Times,* Mar. 28, 1994, A1.

13. H. Meyer, "Breast Study Woes Preview Reform Barriers," *American Medical News,* Mar. 8, 1993, 1.

14. L. K. Stell, "Stopping Treatment on Grounds of Futility: A Role for Institutional Policy," *St. Louis University Public Law Review* 11, no. 2 (1992): 481–97, at 489.

15. *In re Quinlan,* 70 N.J. 10, 355 A.2d 647 (1976).

16. A. Meisel, "Legal Myths about Terminating Life Support," *Archives of Internal Medicine* 151 (1991): 1498–1502.

17. M. B. Kapp, "'Cookbook' Medicine: A Legal Perspective," *Archives of Internal Medicine* 150 (1990): 496–500, at 497.

18. Nelson and Cranford, "Legal Advice," 321.

19. S. V. McCrary, J. W. Swanson, H. S. Perkins, and W. J. Winslade, "Treatment Decisions for Terminally Ill Patients: Physicians' Legal Defensiveness and Knowledge of Medical Law," *Law, Medicine, and Health Care* 20, no. 4 (1992): 364–76.

20. *Barber v. Los Angeles County Superior Court,* 195 Cal. Rptr. 484,147 Cal. App. 3d 1006 (1983).

21. *In re Jobes,* 529 A.2d 434 (N.J. 1987).

22. See note 17 above.

23. L. J. Schneiderman, R. A. Pearlman, R. M. Kaplan, et al., "Relationship of General Advance Directive Instructions to Specific Life-Sustaining Treatment Preferences in Patients with Serious Illness," *Archives of Internal Medicine* 152 (1992): 2114–22.

24. At the time of this writing, Georgia, Illinois, and Nevada had statutes (modeled after a California advance directive provision, since re-
scinded) that allow persons completing a "directive to physicians" to request that every possible treatment be employed in the event they become
incompetent, whether or not a treatment is beneficial or futile. Thus, a
patient in Nevada could direct: "I desire that my life be prolonged to the
greatest extent possible, without regard to my condition, the chances I have
for recovery or long-term survival, or the costs of the procedures" (Durable
Power of Attorney for Health Care. Nev. Rev. Sta. Ann 449. 800, 1993). The
practical effect of these statutes remains to be seen. However, they may dis-
courage health providers in these states who seek to practice responsible
medicine (including providing comfort care) rather than pursuing futile life-
prolongation in dying patients.

We have already described in Chapter 4 the issues brought to court in
the case of Helga Wanglie, wherein the family, claiming that a miracle
might occur, demanded aggressive life support of an irrevocably unconscious woman. And as noted already in Chapter 5, the most notorious example of the court being called upon to force medicine to seek a miracle is
In the Matter of Baby K (see also Chapter 10). Baby K was born in October
1992 at Fairfax Hospital in Falls Church, Virginia, with a condition known
as anencephaly, a congenital absence of most of the brain. The vast majority
of infants with anencephaly die within a few days; none ever develops anything remotely resembling consciousness. Rather than allow the infant to
die peacefully, however, the physicians put her on a ventilator, even though
they considered the treatment medically futile. The mother disagreed, and
insisted that all life-prolonging treatments be continued. The child was
moved to a nursing home, but was brought back to the hospital several
times for treatment when she manifested breathing difficulties. After the
child had survived some seventeen months, the hospital finally went to
court for permission to refuse to aggressively treat the child if she returned
again, arguing that the very nature of anencephaly rendered such treatment
futile. The hospital lost in District Court and again in the U.S. Court of
Appeals by a 2 to 1 vote. The appeals court panel invoked the Emergency
Medical Treatment and Active Labor Act, an anti-dumping law intended to
protect seriously ill patients from being dangerously kicked out of emergency facilities because of financial considerations—a move that in this case
was inappropriate, since all the child's hospital bills are being paid for by
Kaiser Permanente, the mother's insurer. The lower court also cited what
lawyer Marshall Kapp calls a legal "wild card," the Americans with Disabilities Act (ADA). Under this civil rights legislation, health care providers, like
other public and private entities, are forbidden to discriminate in the ser-

vices they provide solely on the basis of a recipient's disability, and are required to make "reasonable accommodations" for the sake of disabled recipients. But, as Kapp points out, "if a particular medical intervention truly is futile, no accommodation the provider might make would qualify the patient to benefit from that intervention, and the ADA should be irrelevant. Nonetheless, little guidance exists yet for interpreting the many, often intentional, ambiguities contained in this new law. It remains to be seen whether patients or surrogates will be able to invoke the ADA, by threat or litigation, to frustrate provider wishes to abate futile care on the grounds of discrimination against the disabled" (M. B. Kapp, "Futile Medical Treatment: A Review of the Ethical Arguments and Legal Holdings," *Journal of General Internal Medicine* 9 [1994]: 170–77). For another excellent discussion of the legal aspects of medical futility, see F. H. Marsh and A. Staver, "Physician Authority for Unilateral DNR Orders," *Journal of Legal Medicine* 12 (1993): 115–65.

CHAPTER 7: ETHICAL IMPLICATIONS OF MEDICAL FUTILITY

1. K. Faber-Langendoen, "Resuscitation of Patients with Metastatic Cancer: Is Transient Benefit Still Futile?" *Archives of Internal Medicine* 151 (1991): 235–39.

2. President's Commission for the Study of Ethical Problems in Medicine and Biomedical and Behavioral Research, *Deciding to Forgo Life-Sustaining Treatment* (Washington, D.C.: Government Printing Office, 1983), 44; American Thoracic Society, Bioethics Task Force, "Withholding and Withdrawing Life-Sustaining Therapy," *Annals of Internal Medicine* 115 (1991): 478–85; Task Force on Ethics of the Society of Critical Care Medicine, "Consensus Report on the Ethics of Forgoing Life-Sustaining Treatments in the Critically Ill," *Critical Care Medicine* 18 (1990): 1436.

3. Hippocratic Oath, in *Ethics in Medicine: Historical Perspective and Contemporary Concerns,* ed. J. S. Reiser, A. J. Dyck, and W. J. Curran (Cambridge: MIT Press, 1977), 5.

4. *Plato: The Collected Dialogues,* ed. E. Hamilton and H. Cairns (Princeton: Princeton University Press, 1964), 262.

5. D. A. Shewmon and C. M. De Giorgio, "Early Prognosis in Anoxic Coma: Reliability and Rationale," *Neurologic Clinics* 7 (1989): 823–43.

6. C. O. Hershey and L. Fisher, "Why Outcome of Cardiopulmonary Resuscitation in General Wards Is Poor," *Lancet,* Jan. 2, 1982, 31–34; S. A. Bedell, T. L. Delbanco, E. F. Cook, and F. H. Epstein, "Survival after Cardiopulmonary Resuscitation in the Hospital," *NEJM* 309 (1983): 569–76.

7. President's Commission, *Deciding to Forgo,* 44.

8. D. Humphrey, *Final Exit* (Eugene, Ore.: Hemlock Society, 1991).

9. President's Commission, *Deciding to Forgo,* 44.

10. Hastings Center, *Guidelines on the Termination of Life-Sustaining Treatment and the Care of the Dying* (Indianapolis: Indiana University Press, 1987), 19.

11. American Medical Association, Council on Ethical and Judicial Affairs, "Guidelines for the Appropriate Use of Do-Not-Resuscitate Orders," *JAMA* 265 (1991): 1870.

12. American Thoracic Society, "Life-Sustaining Therapy," 481.

13. Task Force on Ethics, "Consensus Report."

14. Society of Critical Care Medicine Ethics Committee, Consensus Statement on the Triage of Critically Ill Patients, 1993.

15. T. E. Finucane, "Life-Prolonging Treatments Late in Life," *Journal of General Internal Medicine* 8 (1993): 399–400.

16. H. K. Beecher, "The Powerful Placebo," *JAMA* 159 (1955): 1602–6; H. Brody and A. Yates, "The Placebo Response," in *Behavior and Medicine,* ed. D. Wedding (St. Louis: Mosby Yearbook, 1990).

17. J. Katz, *The Silent World of Doctor and Patient* (New York: Free Press, 1984).

18. M. Battin, "Voluntary Euthanasia and the Risk of Abuse: Can We Learn Anything from the Netherlands?" *Law, Medicine, and Health Care* 20 (1992): 133–43, at 137.

19. J. W. Walters, *What Is a Person? Brain Function and Moral Status* (Champaign: University of Illinois Press, in press).

20. J. T. Noonan, Jr., "Development in Moral Doctrine," *Theological Studies* 54 (1993): 662–77, at 669.

21. C. Curran, *Catholic Moral Theology in Dialogue* (Notre Dame: Fides Publishers, 1972), 168–69, at 168.

22. *McNeil/Lehrer News Hour,* Aug. 12, 1993.

23. J. Reitman, personal communication.

24. Ibid.

25. F. Rosner and J. D. Bleich, *Jewish Bioethics* (New York: Hebrew Publishing Co., 1979), 263, 264.

26. B. F. Herring, *Jewish Ethics and Halakah for Our Time* (New York: Yeshiva University Press, 1984), 71; A. Steinberg, "A Jewish Perspective on the Four Principles," in *Principles of Health Care Ethics,* ed. R. Gillon (New York: John Wiley and Sons, 1994).

27. Noonan, "Moral Doctrine," 677.

28. See note 26 above.

CHAPTER 8: THE WAY IT IS NOW / THE WAY IT OUGHT TO BE: FOR PATIENTS

1. *In the Matter of Westchester County Medical Center, on Behalf of Mary O'Connor,* 72 N.Y.2d 517, 531 N.E.2d 607, 534 N.Y.S.2d 886 (1988).

2. S. H. Wanzer, D. D. Federman, and S. J. Adelstein, et al., "The Physician's Responsibility toward Hopelessly Ill Patients: A Second Look," *NEJM* 320 (1989): 844–49; L. J. Schneiderman and R. G. Spragg, "Ethical Decisions in Discontinuing Mechanical Ventilation," *NEJM* 318 (1988): 984–88; M. Angell, "The Quality of Mercy," *NEJM* 306 (1982): 98–99; B. Lo, F. Rouse, and L. Dornbrand, "Family Decision-Making on Trial: Who Decides for Incompetent Patients?" *NEJM* 322 (1990): 1228–31.

3. *In re O'Conner,* 72 N.Y. 2d 517 at 533, 531 N.E. 2d 607 at 615, 534 N.Y.S. 2d 886 at 894.

4. Ibid., 72 N.Y. 2d 517 at 544, 531 N.E. 2d 607 at 622, 534 N.Y.S. 2d 886 at 901.

5. R. M. Dworkin, *Life's Dominion* (New York: Alfred A. Knopf, 1993).

6. R. J. Blendon, U. S. Szalay, and R. A. Knox, "Should Physicians Aid Their Patients in Dying?" *JAMA* 267 (1992): 2658–62.

7. *In re O'Connor,* 72 N.Y. 2d 517 at 551, 531 N.E. 2d 607 at 626, 534 N.Y.S. 2d 886 at 905.

8. D. Callahan, "Medical Futility, Medical Necessity: The Problem without a Name," *Hastings Center Report* July/Aug. (1991): 34.

9. D. Yankelovich, *Coming to Public Judgment: Making Democracy Work in a Complex World* (Syracuse: Syracuse University Press, 1991), 5.

10. Ibid.

11. Ibid., 5, 28.

12. B. Jennings, "Possibilities of Consensus: Toward Democratic Moral Discourse," *Journal of Medicine and Philosophy* 16 (1991): 462.

13. Yankelovich, *Coming to Public Judgment,* 75.

14. Ibid., 65.

15. D. M. Mirvis, " Physicians' Autonomy: The Relation between Public and Professional Expectations," *NEJM* 328 (1993): 1346–49.

16. N. S. Jecker and L. J. Schneiderman, "An Ethical Analysis of the Use of 'Futility' in the 1992 AHA Guidelines for CPR and ECC," *Archives of Internal Medicine* 153 (1993): 2195–98.

17. M. Z. Solomon, L. O'Donnell, and B. Jennings, "Decisions Near the End of Life: Professional Views on Life-Sustaining Treatments," *American Journal of Public Health* 83 (1993): 14–23.

18. L. Edelstein, "The Hippocratic Physician," in *Ancient Medicine: Selected Papers of Ludwig Edelstein,* ed. O. Temkin and C. L. Temkin (Baltimore: Johns Hopkins Press, 1967), 106.

19. Yankelovich, *Coming to Public Judgment,* 240.

CHAPTER 9: THE WAY IT IS NOW / THE WAY IT OUGHT TO BE:
FOR HEALTH PROFESSIONALS

1. W. A. Knaus, D. P. Wagner, E. A. Draper, J. E. Zimmerman, M. Bergner, P. G. Bastos, et al., "The APACHE III Prognostic System: Risk Prediction of Hospital Mortality for Critically Ill Hospitalized Adults," *Chest* 100 (1991): 1619–36; W. A. Knaus, D. P. Wagner, and J. Lynn, "Short-Term Mortality Predictions for Critically Ill Hospitalized Adults: Science and Ethics," *Science* 254 (1991): 389–94; W. A. Knaus, D. P. Wagner, J. E. Zimmerman, and E. A. Draper, "Variations in Mortality and Length of Stay in Intensive Care Units," *Annals of Internal Medicine* 118 (1993): 753–61.

2. R. Macklin, *Enemies of Patients* (New York: Oxford University Press, 1993).

3. J. B. McKinlay, "From Promising Report to Standard Procedure: Seven Stages in the Career of a Medical Innovation," *Milbank Memorial Fund Quarterly Health and Society* 59, no. 3 (1981): 374–411, at 383.

4. *Grace Plaza of Great Neck, Inc. v. Elbaum*, 183, AD 2d 10, 588 NYS 2d 853 (1992).

5. D. M. Eddy, "Medicine, Money, and Mathematics," *American College of Surgery Bulletin* 77 (1992): 36–49, at 41, 43.

6. D. A. Grimes, "Technology Follies," *JAMA* 269 (1993): 3030–32, at 3030.

7. S. C. Schoenbaum, "Towards Fewer Procedures and Better Outcomes," *JAMA* 269 (1993): 794–96, at 795.

8. S. Miles, "Medical Futility," *Law, Medicine, and Health Care* 20, no. 4 (1992): 310–15, at 312.

9. L. K. Altman, "Drug Mixture Curbs HIV in Lab, Doctors Report, But Urge Caution," *New York Times*, Feb. 18, 1993, A1.

10. T. C. Chalmers, "Ethical Aspects of Clinical Trials," *American Journal of Opthalmology* 79 (1975): 753–58.

11. Ibid., 755.

12. M. Z. Solomon et al., "Decisions Near the End of Life: Professional Views of Life-Sustaining Treatments," *American Journal of Public Health* 82 (1993): 14–25.

13. J. M. Wilkinson, "Moral Distress in Nursing Practice: Experience and Effect," *Nursing Forum* 23, no. 1 (1987–88): 16–28, at 20–21.

14. Chalmers, "Ethical Aspects," 754–55.

15. "University Group Diabetes Program: A Study of the Effects of Hypoglycemic Agents on Vascular Complications in Patients with Adult-Onset Diabetes," *Diabetes* 19, suppl. 2 (1970): 747; P. H. Wang, J. Lau, and T. C. Chalmers, "Meta-analysis of Effects of Intensive Blood-Glucose Con-

trol on Late Complications of Type I Diabetes," *Lancet* 341 (1993): 1306–9; Diabetes Control and Complications Trial Research Group, "The Effect of Intensive Treatment of Diabetes on the Development and Progression of Long-Term Complications in Insulin-dependent Diabetes Mellitus," *NEJM* 329 (1993): 977–86; P. Reichard, B. Nilsson, and U. Rosenquist, "The Effect of Long-Term Intensified Insulin Treatment on the Development of Micro-vascular Complications of Diabetes Mellitus," *NEJM* 329 (1993): 304–9.

16. Schoenbaum, "Towards Fewer Procedures," 796.

17. Ibid.

18. G. A. Diamond and T. A. Denton, "Alternative Perspectives on the Biased Foundations of Medical Technology Assessment," *Annals of Internal Medicine* 118 (1993): 455–64.

19. D. Gesensway, "Building a Better Clinical Practice Guideline: Conquering Bias Remains a Key Challenge," *ACP Observer* 13, no. 6 (1993): 1.

20. B. G. Charlton, "Public Health Medicine: A Different Kind of Ethics?" *Journal of the Royal Society of Medicine* 86 (1993): 194–95, at 194.

21. Schoenbaum, "Towards Fewer Procedures," 796.

22. L. J. Schneiderman, R. M. Kaplan, R. A. Pearlman, and H. Teetzel, "Do Physicians' Own Preferences for Life-Sustaining Treatment Influence Their Perceptions of Patients' Preferences?" *Journal of Clinical Ethics* 4 (1993): 28–33.

23. R. F. Uhlmann, R. A. Pearlman, and K. C. Cain, "Physicians' and Spouses' Predictions of Elderly Patients' Resuscitation Preferences," *Journal of Gerontology* 43, no. 5 (1988): 115–21.

24. See note 21 above.

25. J. F. Kasper, A. G. Mulley, and J. E. Wennberg, "Developing Shared Decision-Making Programs to Improve the Quality of Health Care," *QRB* 18 (1992): 183–90.

26. A. Langer, quoted in G. Kolata, "Mammogram Debate Moving from Test's Merits to Its Cost," *New York Times,* Dec. 27, 1993, A1.

27. A. Meisel, "Legal Consensus about Forgoing Life-Sustaining Treatment: Its Status and Its Prospects," *Kennedy Institute of Ethics Journal* 2 (1992): 309–45, at 333.

28. E. Eckholm, "Those Who Pay Health Costs Think about Drawing Lines," *New York Times,* Mar. 28, 1993, sec. 4, p. 1.

29. J. E. Brody, "Personal Health: The Rights of a Dying Patient Are Often Misunderstood, Even by Medical Professionals," *New York Times,* Jan. 27, 1993, B7.

30. D. M. Mirvis, "Physicians' Autonomy: The Relation between Public and Professional Expectations," *NEJM* 328 (1993): 1346–49 at 1347.

31. J. D. Lantos, P. A. Singer, R. M. Walker, et al., "The Illusion of

Futility in Clinical Practice," *American Journal of Medicine* 87 (1989): 81–84; T. Brennan, "Right-to-Die Dilemma: Are Ethics Committees Equipped to Fill Their Roles?" *American Medical News,* Nov. 11 (1991): 28; A. M. Capron, "In Re Helga Wanglie," *Hastings Center Report* Sept./Oct. (1991): 26–28; D. Callahan, "Medical Futility, Medical Necessity: The Problem-without-a-Name," *Hastings Center Report* July/Aug. (1991): 30–35, respectively.

32. President's Commission for the Study of Ethical Problems in Medicine and Biomedical and Behavioral Research, *Deciding to Forgo Life-Sustaining Treatment: Ethical, Medical, and Legal Issues in Treatment Decisions* (Washington, D.C.: Government Printing Office, 1983); *Guidelines on the Termination of Life-Sustaining Treatment and the Care of the Dying* (Briarcliff Manor, N.Y.: Hastings Center, 1987); Council on Ethical and Judicial Affairs, *Current Opinions* (Chicago: Council on Ethical and Judicial Affairs of the American Medical Association, 1989); Task Force on Ethics of the Society of Critical Care Medicine, "Consensus Report on the Ethics of Forgoing Life-Sustaining Treatments in the Critically Ill," *Critical Care Medicine* 18 (1989): 1435–39; American Thoracic Society, "Withholding and Withdrawing Life-Sustaining Therapy," *Annals of Internal Medicine* 115 (1991): 478–85.

33. N. S. Jecker and L. J. Schneiderman, "Futility and Rationing," *American Journal of Medicine* 92 (1992): 189–96.

34. President's Commission for the Study of Ethical Problems in Medicine and Biomedical and Behavioral Research, *Defining Death* (Washington, D.C.: Government Printing Office, 1981); "Guidelines for the Determination of Death," *JAMA* 246 (1981): 2184–86.

35. D. Rennie and A. Flanagin, "Publication Bias: The Triumph of Hope over Experience," *JAMA* 267 (1992): 411–12.

36. Knaus, "APACHE III Prognostic Risk System"; Knaus et al., "Variations in Mortality and Length of Stay"; M. M. Pollack, U. E. Ruttimann, and P. R. Getson, "The Pediatric RISK of Mortality (PRISM) Score," *Critical Care Medicine* 16 (1988): 1110–16; R.W.S. Chang, "Individual Outcome Prediction Models for Intensive Care Units," *Lancet* 2, no. 8655 (1989): 143–46; U. E. Ruttimann and M. M. Pollack, "Objective Assessment of Changing Mortality Risks in Pediatric Intensive Care Unit Patients," *Critical Care Medicine* 19 (1991): 474–83; U. E. Ruttimann and M. M. Pollack, "A Time-Series Approach to Outcome Prediction," *Computers and Biomedical Research* 26 (1993): 353–72.

37. L. J. Schneiderman, N. S. Jecker, and A. R. Jonsen, "Medical Futility: Its Meaning and Ethical Implications," *Annals of Internal Medicine* 112 (1990): 949–54.

38. Emergency Cardiac Care Committee and Subcommittees, American Heart Association, "Guidelines for Cardiopulmonary Resuscitation

and Emergency Cardiac Care, VII: Ethical Considerations in Resuscitation," *JAMA* 268 (1992): 2282–88; N. S. Jecker and L. J. Schneiderman, "Ceasing Futile Resuscitation in the Field: Ethical Considerations," *Archives of Internal Medicine* 152 (1992): 2392–97; N. S. Jecker and L. J. Schneiderman, "An Ethical Analysis of the Use of 'Futility' in the 1992 American Heart Association Guidelines for Cardiopulmonary Resuscitation and Emergency Cardiac Care," *Archives of Internal Medicine* 153 (1993): 2195–98; K. M. McIntyre, "Loosening Criteria for Withholding Prehospital Cardiopulmonary Resuscitation," *Archives of Internal Medicine* 153 (1993): 2189–92.

39. J. H. King, *The Law of Medical Malpractice in a Nutshell* (St. Paul: West Publishing Co., 1977), 42–49; J. H. King, "In Search of a Standard of Care for the Medical Profession: The 'Accepted Practice' Formula," *Vanderbilt Law Review* 28 (1975): 1213–76; King, *Law of Medical Malpractice,* 44, 46.

40. M. B. Kapp, "'Cookbook'" Medicine: A Legal Perspective," *Archives of Internal Medicine* 150 (1990): 496–500.

41. L. K. Stell, "Stopping Treatment on Grounds of Futility: A Role for Institutional Policy," *St. Louis University Public Law Review* 11, no. 2 (1992): 481–97.

42. See note 37 above.

43. A. L. Kellerman, D. R. Staves, and B. B. Hackman, "In-Hospital Resuscitation Following Unsuccessful Prehospital Advanced Cardiac Life Support: 'Heroic Efforts' or an Exercise in Futility?" *Annals of Emergency Medicine* 17, no. 6 (1988): 589–94; J. D. Lantos, S. H. Miles, M. D. Silverstein, and C. B. Stocking, "Survival after Cardiopulmonary Resuscitation in Babies of Very Low Birthweight: Is CPR Futile?" *NEJM* 318 (1988): 91–95; G. E. Taffet, T. A. Teasdale, and R. J. Luchi, "In-Hospital Cardiopulmonary Resuscitation," *JAMA* 260 (1988): 2069–72; D. J. Murphy, A. M. Murray, B. E. Robinson, and E. W. Campion, "Outcomes of Cardiopulmonary Resuscitation in the Elderly," *Annals of Internal Medicine* 111 (1989): 199–205; M. J. Bonnin and R. A. Swor, "Outcomes in Unsuccessful Field Resuscitation Attempts," *Annals of Emergency Medicine* 18, no. 5 (1989): 507–12; K. Faber-Langendoen, "Resuscitation of Patients with Metastatic Cancer: Is Transient Benefit Still Futile?" *Archives of Internal Medicine* 151 (1991): 235–39; W. A. Gray, R. J. Capone, and A. S. Most, "Unsuccessful Emergency Medical Resuscitation: Are Continued Efforts in the Emergency Department Justified?" *NEJM* 329 (1991): 1393–98.

44. D. J. Murphy and T. E. Finucane, "New Do-Not-Resuscitate Policies: A First Step in Cost Control," *Archives of Internal Medicine* 153 (1993): 1641–48.

45. M. Rosenberg, C. Wang, S. Hoffman-Wilde, and D. Hickham, "Results of Cardiopulmonary Resuscitation: Failure to Predict Survival in

Two Community Hospitals," *Archives of Internal Medicine* 153 (1993): 1370–75.

46. K. M. McIntyre, "Failure of 'Predictors' of Cardiopulmonary Resuscitation Outcomes to Predict Cardiopulmonary Resuscitation Outcomes," ibid., 1293–96.

47. L. J. Schneiderman and N. S. Jecker, "Futility in Practice," *Archives of Internal Medicine* 153 (1993): 437–41.

48. "At Odds with Family, Hospital Seeks to End Life," *Chicago Tribune*, Jan. 10, 1991; "Atlanta Court Bars Efforts to End Life Support for Stricken Girl, 13," *New York Times*, Oct. 18, 1991; Gianelli, "Hospital Seeks to Override Family's Objections, Stop Respirator," *American Medical News*, Jan. 28, 1992, sec. 2; Belkin, "As Family Protests, Hospital Seeks an End to Woman's Life Support," *New York Times*, Jan. 10, 1991, A1.

49. *In the Matter of Baby "K,"* U.S. Court of Appeals for the Fourth Circuit: no. 93–1899; no. 93–1923; no. 93–1924.

CHAPTER 10: SUMMING UP: MEDICAL FUTILITY

1. *In the Matter of Baby "K,"* U.S. Court of Appeals for the Fourth Circuit: no. 93–1899; no. 93–1923; no. 93–1924.

2. Public Law No. 101–336 (July 26, 1990).

3. L. J. Schneiderman, N. S. Jecker, and A. R. Jonsen, "Medical Futility: Its Meaning and Ethical Implications," *Annals of Internal Medicine* 112, no. 12 (1990): 949–54.

4. J. D. Lantos, P. A. Singer, R. M. Walter, et al., "The Illusion of Futility in Clinical Practice," *American Journal of Medicine* 87 (1989): 81–84; S. J. Youngner, "Who Defines Futility?" *JAMA* 260 (1988): 2094–95.

5. J. J. Paris, M. D. Schreiber, M. Statter, R. Arensman, and M. Siegler, "Beyond Autonomy: Physicians' Refusal to Use Life-Prolonging Extracorporeal Membrane Oxygenation," *NEJM* 329 (1993): 354–57, at 356.

6. D. W. Amundsen, "The Physician's Obligation to Prolong Life: A Medical Duty without Classical Roots," *Hastings Center Report* 8, no. 4 (1978): 23–30.

7. R. D. Truog, A. S. Brett, and J. Frader, "The Problem with Futility," *NEJM* 326 (1992): 1560–64.

8. President's Commission for the Study for Ethical Problems in Medicine and Biomedical and Behavioral Research, *Deciding to Forgo Life-Sustaining Treatment: Ethical, Medical, and Legal Issues in Treatment Decisions* (Washington, D.C.: Government Printing Office, 1983); *Guidelines on the Termination of Life-Sustaining Treatment and the Care of the Dying* (Briarcliff Manor, N.Y.: Hastings Center, 1987); Council on Ethical and Judicial Affairs, *Current Opinions* (Chicago: Council on Ethical and Judicial Affairs

of the American Medical Association, 1989); Task Force on Ethics of the Society of Critical Care Medicine, "Consensus Report on the Ethics of For-going Life-Sustaining Treatments in the Critically Ill," *Critical Care Medicine* 18 (1990): 1435–39; American Thoracic Society, "Withholding and With-drawing Life-Sustaining Therapy," *Annals of Internal Medicine* 115 (1991): 478–85.

9. See note 7.

10. D. Postema, Personal communication.

11. Hippocratic corpus, "The Art," in *Ethics in Medicine: Historical Per-spectives and Contemporary Concerns,* ed. S. J. Reiser, A. J. Dyck, and W. J. Cur-ran (Cambridge: MIT Press, 1977), pp. 6–7.

12. Plato, in *Republic,* trans. G.M.A. Grube (Indianapolis: Hackett Publishing Co., 1981), pp. 76–77.

13. A. L. Kellermann, D. R. Staves, and B. B. Hackman, "In-Hospital Resuscitation Following Unsuccessful Prehospital Advanced Cardiac Life-Support: 'Heroic Efforts' or an Exercise in Futility?" *Annals of Emergency Medicine* 17, no. 6 (1988): 589–94; J. D. Lantos, S. H. Miles, M. D. Silverstein, and C. B. Stocking, "Survival after Cardiopulmonary Resuscitation in Babies of Very Low Birth Weight: Is CPR Futile?" *NEJM* 318 (1988): 91–95; G. E. Taffet, T. A. Teasdale, and R. J. Luchi, "In-Hospital Cardiopulmo-nary Resuscitation," *JAMA* 260 (1988): 2069–72; D. J. Murphy, A. M. Mur-ray, B. E. Robinson, et al., "Outcomes of Cardiopulmonary Resuscitation in the Elderly," *Annals of Internal Medicine* 111 (1989): 199–205; M. J. Bonnin and R. A. Swor, "Outcomes in Unsuccessful Field Resuscitation Attempts," *Annals of Emergency Medicine* 18, no. 5 (1989): 507–12; K. Faber-Langendoen, "Resuscitation of Patients with Metastatic Cancer: Is Transient Benefit Still Futile?" *Archives of Internal Medicine* 151 (1991): 235–39; W. A. Gray, R. J. Capone, and A. S. Most, "Unsuccessful Emergency Medical Resuscitation: Are Continued Efforts in the Emergency Department Justified?" *NEJM* 329 (1991): 1393–98.

14. See note 3 above.

15. See note 13 above.

16. N. S. Jecker and L. J. Schneiderman, "Medical Futility: The Duty Not to Treat," *Cambridge Quarterly of Healthcare Ethics* 2 (1993): 151–57.

17. T. Tomlinson and H. Brody, "Futility and the Ethics of Resuscita-tion," *JAMA* 264, no. 10 (1990): 1276–80.

18. See note 7 above.

19. L. J. Schneiderman and N. S. Jecker, "Futility in Practice," *Archives of Internal Medicine* 153 (1993): 437–41.

20. N. S. Jecker and L. J. Schneiderman, "Futility and Rationing," *American Journal of Medicine* 92 (1992): 189–96.

21. L. J. Schneiderman, K. Faber-Langendoen, and N. S. Jecker, "Beyond Futility to an Ethic of Care," *American Journal of Medicine* 96 (1994): 110–14.

22. D. Callahan, "Medical Futility, Medical Necessity: The Problem-without-a-Name," *Hastings Center Report* 21, no. 4 (1991): 30–35, at 34.

23. D. Callahan, letter dated March 1, 1993.

24. A. M. Capron, "In re Helga Wanglie," *Hastings Center Report* 21, no. 5 (1991): 26–28, at 28.

25. See note 7 above.

26. Ibid.

27. See note 19 above.

Library of Congress Cataloging-in-Publication Data

Schneiderman, L. J.
    Wrong medicine : doctors, patients, and futile treatment /
Lawerence J. Schneiderman and Nancy S. Jecker.
        p.   cm.
    Includes bibliographical references and index.
    ISBN 0-8018-5036-3
    1. Medical ethics.   2. Surgery, Unnecessary.   3. Medicine—
Decision making.   I. Jecker, Nancy Ann Silbergeld.   II. Title.
R724.S3936 1995
610.69'6—dc20   94-38799
                                                                CIP